# Download Your Included Ebook Today!

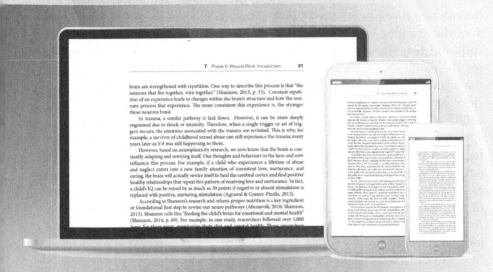

Your print purchase of *Cardiac Diagnosis for Acute Care* **includes an ebook download** to the device of your choice—increasing accessibility, portability, and searchability!

**Download your ebook today at
http://spubonline.com/cardiac
and enter the activation code below:**

BT1N29FPCP

SPRINGER PUBLISHING COMPANY

**Leslie E. Janik, MSN, ARNP, ACNP-BC**, is an instructor of medicine in the College of Medicine, Mayo Clinic, Jacksonville, Florida. She has been a board-certified acute care nurse practitioner in the division of cardiovascular diseases at Mayo Clinic since 2005, when she helped establish a cardiovascular inpatient service. She works closely with the fellowship and residency programs and has assisted in developing protocols for the cardiology hospital and clinic practice. Ms. Janik is also part of the administrative team within her department and is supervisor to the cardiovascular advanced practice providers. She received her BSN from Millikin University in Decatur, Illinois, and her MSN with an acute care specialization from the University of Florida. Her nursing experience included neurology, heart and lung transplantation, and cardiology. In addition to her current role in cardiology, she has worked as an acute care nurse practitioner in both neurology and plastic surgery. She is a member of the Chest Pain Committee at Mayo Clinic, Florida, the American Academy of Nurse Practitioners, and has been published in the online journal *Advance for NPs & PAs*.

# Cardiac Diagnosis for Acute Care

## The NP's and PA's Guide to a Comprehensive History and Deciphering the Differential

*Leslie E. Janik, MSN, ARNP, ACNP-BC*

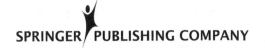

SPRINGER PUBLISHING COMPANY

Springer Publishing Company, LLC
11 West 42nd Street
New York, NY 10036
www.springerpub.com

*Acquisitions Editor*: Elizabeth Nieginski
*Senior Production Editor*: Kris Parrish
*Compositor*: diacriTech, Chennai

*ISBN*: 978-0-8261-4126-2
*ebook ISBN*: 978-0-8261-4143-9

18 19 20 21 / 5 4 3 2 1

The author and the publisher of this Work have made every effort to use sources believed to be reliable to provide information that is accurate and compatible with the standards generally accepted at the time of publication. Because medical science is continually advancing, our knowledge base continues to expand. Therefore, as new information becomes available, changes in procedures become necessary. We recommend that the reader always consult current research and specific institutional policies before performing any clinical procedure. The author and publisher shall not be liable for any special, consequential, or exemplary damages resulting, in whole or in part, from the readers' use of, or reliance on, the information contained in this book. The publisher has no responsibility for the persistence or accuracy of URLs for external or third-party Internet websites referred to in this publication and does not guarantee that any content on such websites is, or will remain, accurate or appropriate.

**Library of Congress Cataloging-in-Publication Data**
Names: Janik, Leslie, author.
Title: Cardiac diagnosis for acute care : the NP's and PA's guide to a
   comprehensive history and deciphering the differential / Leslie Janik.
Description: New York, NY : Springer Publishing Company, LLC, [2018] |
   Includes bibliographical references and index.
Identifiers: LCCN 2017052268 | ISBN 9780826141262 | ISBN 9780826141439 (ebook)
Subjects: | MESH: Diagnostic Techniques, Cardiovascular | Acute Coronary
   Syndrome—diagnosis | Medical History Taking—methods | Diagnosis,
   Differential | Case Reports
Classification: LCC RC670 | NLM WG 141 | DDC 616.1/075—dc23
LC record available at https://lccn.loc.gov/2017052268.

Contact us to receive discount rates on bulk purchases.
We can also customize our books to meet your needs.
For more information please contact: sales@springerpub.com

Printed in the United States of America.

*To my friends and family . . . Without your love, support, and encouragement this would not have been possible.*

*To the reader . . .*
*An inquisitive mind leads to limitless finds.*

# CONTENTS

## PART I: COMMON PRESENTATIONS OF ACUTE CARDIAC CONDITIONS

## PART II: UNCOMMON PRESENTATIONS OF ACUTE CARDIAC CONDITIONS

## PART III: SUMMARY AND USEFUL CLINICAL TOOLS

# FOREWORD

As a physician assistant for more than 23 years who has worked in geriatrics, internal medicine, minimally invasive surgery, women's health, bariatric surgery, and transplant surgery and medicine, I am honored to write this Foreword for my colleague, Leslie Janik. When I request a consultation from Leslie, she not only performs the consult, but also takes the time to explain her decision-making techniques. When I call her, I know I will come away with at least one nugget of knowledge to add to my practitioner toolkit.

Leslie Janik is the ideal person to write this book because of her vast experience in cardiology, her willingness to teach, and her commitment to share her knowledge. My first thought in reviewing this book was, *"It's about time someone wrote a practical, real-life book for advanced practice providers!"* This book should have been written years ago, and I am excited to share it with my students and physician assistant colleagues. With *Cardiac Diagnosis for Acute Care,* providers now have a *practical* guide to use when caring for patients who present in various settings with cardiac complaints.

This book prepares new providers in acute care settings to ask the right questions, ask questions early, immediately begin to form a differential diagnosis, and take the best care of the patient who presents with chest pain, shortness of breath, and syncope. Leslie's book is a must-read for all physician assistants and nurse practitioners who need a handy tool to meet the needs of their patients when they enter the acute care setting.

The case scenario format, contrasting the history obtained by an emergency department provider from that of a cardiovascular provider, helps readers identify critical findings simply and clearly. Leslie's care in highlighting components of the history prepares the reader to begin to formulate a differential diagnosis early, and with ease. The inclusion of key features and the comparison and analysis of histories help readers to improve their clinical acumen. Leslie does not stop there; she goes on to explain each differential diagnosis. These features combine to make this cardiology handbook an essential reference for providers in acute care settings.

Leslie's process, in focusing on key features of the history, physical exam, and other assessment findings, and the ability to put it all together, is analogous to working out a problem—you cannot wait to get to the answer to see if you are right. I was impressed by her case scenarios and surprised by the uncommon presentations of acute cardiac conditions. This is the only book for providers that breaks down troponins in a way you will not forget! The lessons on fatigue, cough, and abdominal pain are invaluable because of the Q&A method used. I am so excited to see this book in print.

Leslie is right: History taking is an art. She not only gives us a practical guide, but also a resource to share with students to help them provide confident care during and after training. She provides a bonus section on writing up complete history and physical examination findings, which is a "must" for everyone, advanced practice student and provider alike. She complements this with a complete consult write-up that gives students and providers the opportunity to see the different lenses specialty providers use in their evaluations.

This book breaks down each problem, supporting you, me, and any provider who treats patients with acute cardiac complaints. This book is exactly what we noncardiology providers need to make us more confident in how we assess a patient who presents with cardiac complaints. I am excited to have been given the opportunity to read it and look forward to promoting a book that is effective in getting the message across to providers in a way that is helpful, practical, and *not boring*.

Thank you, Leslie.

*Susan M. Salahshor, PhD, PA-C DFAAPA*
*Lead Physician Assistant, Abdominal Transplant*
*Mayo Clinic, Jacksonville, Florida*
*President, Florida Academy of Physician Assistants (2017–2018)*

# FOREWORD

In her conclusion to this book, Leslie Janik likens the acquisition of the medical history to a work of art, in which multiple components must come together to create a whole. I might enlarge on this notion by suggesting likeness also to creating good music—the key to which is practice, practice, practice. As with a learned piece of music, a specific history, heard once, is embedded in memory to be called up when heard again, as the need arises. For clinicians early in their careers, it is essential not only to learn which questions to ask, as is so brilliantly conveyed in this book, but also how to interpret information volunteered after the initial "How can I help you?" or similar opening. Finding the optimum mixture of silence with listening and observation of body language, redirecting and listening, double checking and listening, and then moving on to complete the history efficiently but accurately are all behaviors that must be learned. In this book, the author exposes key questions and lines of questioning systematically for the most common complaints for which hospital-based cardiologists are consulted—chest pain, acute dyspnea, syncope, and troponin elevation, among others—and highlights and discusses both typical and atypical presentations of important conditions in which an accurate history, exam, and subsequent action are key to the best possible outcome for the patient.

Exposure to the acute care cardiac patient requires sacrifices: irregular schedules, time away from family, sleep disruption, and so on. Since our practice added advanced care practitioners in 2005, Leslie Janik has functioned in this role, the last several years as supervisor, so her cumulative exposure to the sorts of histories presented is truly massive. It has been my great fortune to watch her grow in her role from mentee to supervisor and colleague. If history taking is similar to playing a musical instrument, she is a virtuoso. Her case scenarios are best read one at a time, ideally when evaluating patients with the same type of complaint. The straightforward methodology of evaluation and consideration of differential diagnoses are playbooks for evaluating patients, and thus a reference for everyday use for practitioners on the frontline. I am reminded of reference materials used early in my own career that I found similarly essential when seeing individual patients—Degowin's *Diagnostic Examination*, the *Washington Manual of Medical Therapeutics*, and the Profiles chapters in Grossman and Bain's *Cardiac Catheterization*—all of which I also would recommend to the contemporary cardiac practitioner.

The payoff from accurate assessment is, of course, the immense satisfaction received by the practitioner in getting a good outcome for the patient. Examples highlighted in the book are immediate relief of dire symptoms with catheter drainage of cardiac tamponade, emergency surgery for acute dissection of the ascending aorta, and thrombolytic therapy of submassive pulmonary embolism. Other examples would include seeing stroke deficits melt away under the influence of thrombolytic therapy, relief of cardiogenic shock by emergent percutaneous coronary angioplasty and stenting in ST-segment elevation myocardial infarction, and relief of agonizing respiratory distress in a patient with acute pulmonary edema with intravenous diuresis, to name but a few.

For those of us later in our careers, this book provides a reminder that history taking is a skill never quite perfected and in need of continuous refreshment, requiring continuing education and an open mind. In my late 50s, I first learned that one third of hypertrophic cardiomyopathy (HCM) patients had a definite post-prandial exacerbation of symptoms, and that 10% to 20% have an acquired bleeding history due to acquired von Willebrand syndrome, which is discussed in this book in the Chapter 8 scenario detailing the patient with aortic endocarditis. So now I ask HCM patients about nosebleeds, gastrointestinal bleeds, and transfusion. Only this year I learned that patients who have had a Nissen fundoplication cannot drink carbonated beverages because they cannot burp effectively. So, never stop listening, reading, learning.

There has been a trend in professional continuing medical education (CME) offerings in recent years away from didactic presentations to case-based learning. While history and exam findings are featured, they tend to be given a back seat to imaging and cutting-edge technology. Upstream of these dazzling and expensive imaging techniques, we have the clinical evaluation, which is increasingly performed by nurse practitioners or physician assistants, supervised by hospitalists or others. Inasmuch as the imaging modalities are widely disseminated, the excellence of any institution might best be defined by the consistency with which frontline physician extenders and physicians make proper initial assessments. This book represents an important "how-to" guide to foster excellence in those assessments.

*Joseph L. Blackshear, MD*
*Consultant in Cardiovascular Diseases*
*Professor of Medicine*
*Mayo Clinic, Jacksonville, Florida*

# PREFACE

Anyone who has been in practice for any length of time has experienced a situation in which a patient tells one provider one thing and a second provider something else. This happens even when the patient is asked the same question by both. These variables can be hard to account for when trying to evaluate a patient. While we may not be able to control the patient's responses, we can control how we ask the questions in order to elicit a clear and consistent response. *That concept is a particular focus of this book.*

Many books and other resources focus on the differential diagnosis, various disease processes, and the appropriate treatment plan for such. However, very little of what has been published discusses the history of a present illness in any great detail, or how important this history is in determining the correct diagnosis.

In the acute care setting, cardiovascular clinicians are asked to evaluate many patients with symptoms that might suggest an acute cardiac diagnosis. We can take into account that patients may change their answers, but often the information presented to us by the first point of contact can be misleading. We are told the patient's presentation and any relevant data along with a suspected diagnosis, about which we are asked to render an opinion. *I have learned in my own practice that there is usually a lot more information we can gather about the complaint by asking more comprehensive questions in a manner that is clear for the patient to understand.*

To get every bit of information about the patient's symptoms, the line of questioning has to be very specific and detailed—dissecting the symptoms down to their core. When this is done effectively, a diagnosis can often be made just by utilizing the history alone. This, in turn, can lead to an accelerated evaluation and treatment and, ultimately, a positive outcome for the patient.

In this book, clinical scenarios are presented that involve various chief complaints and reasons for consults that typically confront cardiovascular clinicians in an acute care setting. These scenarios will challenge you to look beyond what seems obvious and to think of atypical presentations of acute cardiac issues. The history that is obtained by two providers is compared and broken down to demonstrate the differences in questioning, and how such differences contribute to differing diagnoses.

The objective is to help the novice and experienced clinician alike—particularly those evaluating patients with potential cardiac problems—identify and extract key features of the chief complaint in order to formulate an accurate diagnosis. By the end of this book you will become proficient in using a streamlined approach when questioning the patient, allowing you to obtain data and formulate a concise, detailed, and thorough history of the present illness.

*Leslie E. Janik*

# Assessment, Diagnosis, and Patient History in Acute Cardiac Presentations

Healthcare providers working in the field of cardiology often encounter patients with critical issues that require prompt evaluation and diagnosis. If an accurate diagnosis is delayed or inadequate information is gathered, it can mean the difference between life and death for the patient. Becoming an expert in this field requires the ability to take a thorough history in a timely fashion, interpret all data, and identify what may be relevant to the chief complaint.

Often, patients present with classic symptoms of a diagnosis, and it is simple to draw a conclusion and initiate treatment. At other times, however, the presentation may not be what it seems. When this happens, a patient may be misdiagnosed, undergoing unnecessary evaluation without any relief of symptoms. *It is the responsibility of every provider to avoid making assumptions. Rather, he or she must dissect the chief complaint to avoid delay and potentially costly workups that may not be indicated.*

All providers learn the basic skills of assessment and diagnosis in their various training programs. It is not until working in a specialty role that we learn the nuances of the assessment and physical exam that are specific to the diagnoses we see most often. As cardiovascular clinicians, we should be well versed in evaluating a patient with chest pain and other chief complaints that we see frequently in our practices. With experience, we learn to dig deeper into the patient's complaint and ask questions other providers might not have thought to ask in order to identify whether the patient is having an acute cardiac issue such as an aortic dissection, acute coronary syndrome, or even a life-threatening arrhythmia. In an acute care setting, cardiovascular clinicians are often called upon to determine the appropriate course of action and treatment with this knowledge in mind.

Diagnosing acute cardiac conditions is challenging but rewarding. Each patient can be viewed as a mystery to be solved, and each piece of information we obtain as a clue to help solve the mystery. As specialists in this role, our focus should be to uncover all the information the patient can provide about the chief complaint. This includes everything about the character of the complaint, the timing, what the patient was feeling before, and whatever else is associated with it. The assessment should include the following:

- The past medical history as well as the other histories need to be carefully reviewed with the patient and any concerns clarified, as much as possible.

- The patient's medications need to be reviewed for compliance and accuracy.

- A thorough cardiovascular exam should include careful auscultation of the lungs and heart, palpation of the chest, assessment of the pulses, and evaluation for any bruits.

- Evaluating the abdomen and extremities is also necessary.

A limited amount of objective data is usually available at the time cardiovascular clinicians initially evaluate these patients. The electrocardiogram (ECG), any labs, and imaging data obtained can be crucial in helping to solidify the working diagnosis developed during the encounter. These elements should come together in such a way that the cardiovascular clinician can make a prompt and accurate diagnosis.

In the current environment of rising healthcare costs and demands placed on providers, we are often required to see more patients and have less time and fewer resources in which to do so. The availability of electronic medical records enables providers to gather a lot of information about past medical history, procedures, and medications when seeing a patient who has previously received care at a particular institution.

These details are often referenced in the admission or consult note to fulfill necessary requirements so staff can move on to the next patient. This information can be very helpful, especially when patients are not able to give an accurate history or provide details about prior procedures.

The existence of this previously archived data can, however, foster complacency. Providers may assume that prior histories and lists of medications are still accurate, which can lead to inappropriate drug therapy or failure to capture an important piece of data that is critical to the patient's plan of care.

Medicolegal aspects must also be considered in the acute care setting. Practice has been geared toward the utilization of costly imaging and testing as well as hospitalization to ensure that a critical diagnosis is not missed, particularly in the emergency department setting. One study examined how medicolegal concerns impacted admission rates of patients presenting with possible acute coronary syndrome. The researchers found that emergency physicians would not have admitted 30% of the cases if there had been a hypothetical medicolegal risk of zero, or a 1% to 2% acceptable miss rate (Booker et al., 2015). A perception of zero medicolegal risk would likely reduce admission rates and expensive testing.

Not every patient with chest pain needs a stress test, CT scan of the chest, or coronary angiography, but providers may fear that without them, a patient may slip through a gap in the diagnostic process and suffer an unwanted outcome. As cardiovascular clinicians, we can aid in determining which patients require this type of testing by utilizing a comprehensive history and objective data collection process.

The field of cardiology encompasses many conditions, both chronic and acute. In the acute care setting, cardiovascular clinicians have an obligation to identify a diagnosis and treatment plan promptly in order to provide the patient with the best possible outcome. Other specialists, as well as emergency department physicians, rely on the expertise we can provide to assist in the best management plan for these patients.

I think many clinicians would agree that the most important piece of information obtained when evaluating the patient is the history. The history is what gives us the story so we can understand why patients sought or were brought for care, how they were feeling, and how we are going to best treat them. A comprehensive history can guide us to a diagnosis before any other data are gathered.

I like to use the analogy of a painting. Let us say you are looking at a painting of a bouquet of flowers. Now think of how you would describe that painting to someone who was not physically present with you or to someone who has lost their sight. If you simply told them what kinds and colors of flowers were included, would that person have a mental picture of what you see? Probably not. In order for them to get an idea of what you are looking at, you would need to describe the background, the vase, the texture, and type of arrangement. You would need to describe every color among the flowers in the bouquet, how many there are, and how they are painted, right? That is similar to the process we use when gathering a history. We want to find out everything about the patient's symptoms in order to paint a clear and detailed picture of why he or she is being evaluated.

You will see throughout this book how very different that picture can appear when painted by two different providers. If each provider asked the same questions and received the same information, should not the pictures match?

In the clinical scenarios used to organize the content of this book, a typical cardiovascular chief complaint is broken down into key features. This process demonstrates how subtle differences in questioning can lead to differences in the history that is presented. In an acute care setting, patients often present with vague complaints that could signify any number of things that can raise concerns of a cardiac cause. Knowing the right questions to ask and what information is missing can enable you to quickly confirm or rule out an acute cardiac diagnosis.

Taking a comprehensive history is an art. The skilled clinician should utilize each key feature of a chief complaint to paint a vivid, masterfully crafted picture that is presented in such a way that others can visualize it without seeing it.

# REFERENCE

Booker, J., Hastings, J., Major-Monfried, H., Maron, C., Winkel, M., Wijeratne, H., ... Newman, E. (2015). The association between medicolegal and professional concerns and chest pain admission rates. *Academic Emergency Medicine*, 22(7), 883–886.

# PART I

# Common Presentations of Acute Cardiac Conditions

In the field of cardiology, certain symptoms are seen more frequently than in many other specialty areas. The common complaints of chest pain, shortness of breath, and syncope are a few of the ones we encounter most often. Often, these complaints are coupled with other symptoms, such as nausea, vomiting, palpitations, or swelling. All it takes is a mix of a good story coupled with a few of those symptoms to equal a possible cardiac issue.

In addition to being consulted about the previously noted symptoms, cardiovascular clinicians are frequently asked to evaluate abnormal electrocardiograms (ECGs) and cardiac biomarkers. Most of our time in an acute care setting is spent assessing patients with these symptoms or abnormal objective findings to determine what, if any, cardiac issue is occurring.

As experts in the field, it is also our job to offer reassurance to both patients and other providers when data do not match the clinical picture, raising concern about a possible underlying cardiac issue. In such cases, we may confirm a suspected diagnosis and pursue the workup and management of the patient's condition. Other times, we offer alternative explanations and provide guidance on how to proceed amid what may be confusing data.

Chapters 1 through 8 illustrate chief complaints through clinical scenarios that are commonly seen in an acute care setting. For each scenario, the history and other data are reviewed and examined to demonstrate how seemingly common cardiac issues may not have a cardiac origin at all. As acute care providers, we spend much of our time in emergency departments evaluating patients for potential acute cardiac issues. We are able to negate or support the clinical suspicion by simply taking a comprehensive history. It is not necessarily the responsibility of an emergency department provider to diagnose and treat a suspected underlying cardiac condition, but rather to know when the data support a potential issue and the need for cardiovascular expertise.

Acute care providers are often consulted with a specific question or concern in mind. Other times, the expertise required of this specialty leads us down a different path altogether—one that may not lead to a cardiac diagnosis.

# CHAPTER 1

# Chest Pain: A First Look

## DEFINITION AND SIGNIFICANCE OF CHEST PAIN

According to *Mosby's Medical Dictionary* (2009), chest pain is defined as "a physical complaint that requires immediate diagnosis and evaluation." Chest pain is a common reason people present to an acute care setting. According to the most recent National Hospital Ambulatory Medical Care Survey in 2013, chest pain accounted for nearly 5% of all emergency department visits, second only to abdominal pain (Rui, Kang, & Albert, 2013).

Most people associate chest pain with heart-related conditions, but in many instances it is related to other causes. In only 30% of patients presenting with chest pain is there a cardiac origin for the pain (Chan, Maurice, Davies, & Walters, 2014). Acute care clinicians need to ask the right questions and review relevant data to determine the nature of the chest pain in a timely manner to avoid a potentially dire outcome for these patients.

This chapter and Chapter 2 present case scenarios that demonstrate how differently the evaluation of chest pain can unfold as the examiner dissects the chief complaint through detailed questioning and review of data.

## CASE SCENARIO

The on-call cardiovascular clinician has been asked to consult on a patient with a complaint of chest pain. The initial history, labeled history A, was obtained by the emergency department provider, a physician. History B was taken by the consulting cardiovascular clinician. The consulting clinician is given the initial information and is also told by the emergency physician that the physical exam was unremarkable for any pertinent findings.

# HISTORY A

*A 69-year-old African American male presents to the emergency department at 1900 with a complaint of <u>chest discomfort with burning</u>. He has a past medical history of hypertension, type 2 diabetes mellitus, hyperlipidemia, and coronary artery disease for which he underwent stenting 4 years ago. The <u>pain occurred at 11 a.m. while he was supine</u>. Pain <u>does not change with movement nor does it radiate</u>. The patient <u>did not take any medication to relieve it</u> but is pain free currently. He had a <u>similar episode 2 days ago in the evening</u>.*

Available data thus far are as follows:

## VITAL SIGNS

*Blood pressure*: 142/84 mmHg

*Pulse*: 70 beats per minute

*Respirations*: 14 breaths per minute

*Oxygen saturation*: 99% on room air

*Temperature*: 36.9°C

(*continued*)

## VITAL SIGNS (*continued*)

### Biomarkers, Lab Results, and Diagnostic Tests

The troponin T level is less than 0.01 ng/mL. The ECG shows no ischemic findings and no change from an ECG performed 6 months earlier (when the patient came to the same institution for a shoulder injury). A D-dimer level, basic chemistry panel, and complete blood count (CBC) are also unremarkable. The chest radiograph is clear.

### Home Medications

These have been documented based on the patient's earlier visit and are as follows: Lisinopril, 20 mg daily; metoprolol, 25 mg daily; aspirin, 81 mg daily; omeprazole, 20 mg daily; metformin, 500 mg twice daily; and atorvastatin, 40 mg daily.

In which direction would this presentation lead you? Does this patient require a cardiac workup or not?

# HISTORY B

*A 69-year-old African American male with multiple cardiovascular risk factors, including known coronary artery disease with prior stenting 4 years ago, presents to the emergency department at 1900 with complaints of chest pain and burning. He describes the pain as more of a mild ache with a burning quality that is epigastric in nature. He noticed it about 11 a.m. while lying down after he just finished a late breakfast. He denies any acid brash (taste) associated with the pain. The pain was nonpleuritic and nonpositional. It was not associated with any nausea, vomiting, or diaphoresis. Nothing he did made the symptoms better or worse. He did not take anything for the symptoms. He stated that the pain waxed and waned for about an hour and went away on its own. He had a similar episode 2 days earlier after eating dinner; however, it did not last as long as his episode today. Both episodes were the same in severity.*

He <u>denies having experienced these symptoms prior to his cardiac stent</u>. At that time, his primary symptom was shortness of breath, which he currently denies. After further questioning the patient relates that he has a history of <u>gastroesophageal reflux disease (GERD)</u> and the only other time he's had similar symptoms is with his "reflux"; however, given his cardiac history he wanted to come in and be sure. <u>Review of medications revealed that the patient has not been taking his omeprazole for 1 week. He was recently started on amlodipine, 5 mg daily, and he was under the impression this medication replaced the omeprazole. When questioned about the absence of ticagrelor or clopidogrel—since he has a history of cardiac stent—he recalls that he took clopidogrel for 2 months after his stent procedure and was told by his cardiologist that he no longer needed anything more than an aspirin after that.</u>

In which direction would this presentation lead you? Cardiac workup or not?

## KEY FEATURES OF THE HISTORY

Key features of the history are those details obtained about the patient's complaint in order to formulate the history. *In both history A and history B, the key points relevant to the chief complaint are underlined.* As providers, we learn to extract six basic features of a chief complaint. Those features are:

1. Character (including location and severity)
2. Timing (including onset)
3. Duration
4. Associated symptoms
5. Mitigating factors
6. Alleviating factors

Both of the histories cover these features, but clearly history B digs more deeply into each one and extracts as much detail as possible. The result is a very different presentation and a different plan of care. Let us break down each feature and identify interview techniques to teach you how to get from A to B.

## Character

The provider in history A identified the character of the chief complaint by asking the patient the following questions:

Q: **What brought you here today?**

A: Discomfort and burning in my chest.

Q: **Have you had this before?**

A: Yes, 2 days ago in the evening.

Q: **Does the pain change with movement or does it radiate?**

A: No.

Now let us look at how the provider in history B questioned the patient about the character of the pain:

Q: **What brought you here today?**

A: Discomfort and burning in my chest.

Q: **Is the discomfort separate from the burning sensation or do they occur together?**

A: They occur together. It's more of a burning than pain.

Q: **Show me where your discomfort and burning is located.**

A: Here. (The patient points to his upper epigastric region.)

Q: **Does the discomfort and burning radiate anywhere—like your arm, jaw, back, or throat?**

A: No, it stays right in that spot for the most part.

Q: **Does the discomfort feel like a pressure sensation? Is it sharp, heavy, stabbing, squeezing, dull, or aching?**

A: It's a very dull ache that I felt with the burning.

Q: **Does it change with movement or deep breathing?**

A: No.

Q: **Did you notice any acid taste in the back of your throat?**

A: No. It feels like my heartburn.

Q: **Have you had this sensation before today?**

A: Yes, 2 days ago.

Q: **Did that episode feel the same as today or was it more severe? Less severe?**

A: It was about the same.

Q: **Did you have these symptoms when you had your cardiac stent placed?**

A: No. It didn't feel anything like this. I only felt short of breath then.

It is important to note that both providers started the conversation with an open-ended question, "What brought you here today?" This is a good technique because it does not allow for any assumptions and it provides insight as to what exactly prompted the patient to seek care.

This approach can be important when patients present with multiple complaints. Often, they are short of breath with chest pain and nausea, so asking them why they came in can identify which symptom, if any, the patient found more concerning. Both providers in these histories also asked why the patient was there, when the pain occurred, and whether or not it radiated. The provider in history B, however, was much more specific and asked about the location and type of discomfort, and whether it was similar to the patient's prior cardiac event. This is a critical question to ask of any patient who has a prior cardiac history since often, but not always, the symptoms are similar to what they experienced in the past.

## Timing and Duration

The provider in history A asks the following questions about the timing and duration of the patient's symptoms:

Q: **What time did you notice the pain?**

A: Around 11 a.m. today.

Q: **What were you doing at the time?**

A: Lying down.

Q: **What time did the episode occur 2 days ago?**

A: In the evening, around 6 p.m.

Here's how the provider in history B obtained information about the timing and duration of symptoms:

Q: **What time did you notice the pain?**

A: Around 11 a.m. today.

Q: **Were you doing anything at the time, such as exerting yourself, eating, or did it occur at rest?**

A: I was lying down when I noticed it. I had just finished eating a late breakfast.

Q: **What time did the episode occur 2 days ago? Was it also after a meal?**

A: It occurred around 6 p.m. Now that you mention it, it did happen after I had eaten dinner.

Q: **How long did the symptoms last today?**

A: They came and went for about an hour.

Q: **Specifically, how long did each episode last within that hour?**

A: About 5 minutes or so.

Q: **Did the episode 2 days ago also wax and wane for an hour with each occurrence also lasting around 5 minutes, or was it shorter?**

A: I think it was about the same, maybe longer.

Again, both providers touched on the basics of timing, but the provider in history A neglected to ask about the duration of the symptoms of both episodes.

If this is truly an acute coronary syndrome, the symptoms progress and worsen in both severity and duration with each occurrence (Giugliano, Cannon, & Braunwald, 2015), which is why it is very important to question the patient specifically about these details, as the provider in history B did. Often providers assume patients will disclose details about their symptoms without prompting, but in many cases, they do not elaborate on their own without being asked specifically. In this case, the patient knew his pain occurred after a meal, but since the first provider did not ask, he may have felt it was not relevant.

## Associated Symptoms

The provider in history A failed to ask the patient about any associated symptoms that might have occurred with the burning and discomfort. The provider in history B asked the following:

Q: **Did you have any nausea, vomiting, sweating, or lightheadedness with these symptoms?**

A: No.

Q: **Have you noticed any shortness of breath, fatigue, or decreased endurance performing usual activities in the past several days or weeks?**

A: No. I have felt well aside from these two episodes.

Given the patient's cardiac history, the provider in history B is trying to determine if there are any relevant associated symptoms, which often accompany unstable angina or acute coronary syndrome. In addition, the patient stated that with his prior cardiac event, his only symptom was shortness of breath, so it is important to ask about that since many times patients have similar symptoms with each event. Many patients, in hindsight, report they felt more fatigued and tired leading up to their cardiac event, but did not associate the two as being related. It is important that the clinician ask about the symptoms in detail, but also all symptoms that might have led to this point, to determine if they could be connected in any way.

## Mitigating or Alleviating Factors

The provider in history A asked the following question about mitigating or alleviating factors:

Q: **Did you take anything for your symptoms before coming in today?**

A: No. Eventually I felt better.

The provider in history B asked these questions related to mitigating or alleviating factors:

Q: **Did you take anything to get rid of the pain?**

A: No.

Q: **Did any position improve or worsen the pain, such as lying down, standing up, or sitting?**

A: No, it did not change with anything I did.

Both providers asked if the patient took anything to make the pain better. In any patient with angina, nitroglycerin often improves the pain. This would be important information to have as you are working up the patient since it would lead your thoughts toward a cardiac diagnosis, although relief with nitroglycerin does not necessarily mean the diagnosis is cardiac (Grailey & Glasziou, 2012). However, if the patient reported he took a TUMS or an antacid and his symptoms improved, this would suggest his symptoms were gastrointestinal in origin. How patients treat their symptoms before arrival in the acute care setting can be extremely helpful in determining the differential diagnosis.

## KEY FEATURES OF THE DATA

The key features of the data include any objective data that might be relevant to the chief complaint, as well as the medication list and relevant histories. In a patient with a chief complaint of chest pain, the key objective features are as follows:

- Vital signs
- ECG
- Chest radiograph
- Biomarkers (such as troponin), D-dimer
- Basic chemistry panel and CBC

These data were available at the time both providers interviewed the patient. Let us break the data down further and discuss each component.

## Vital Signs

The following findings were reported:

*Blood pressure*: 142/84 mmHg

*Pulse*: 70 beats per minute

*Respirations*: 14 breaths per minute

*Oxygen saturation*: 99% on room air

*Temperature*: 36.9°C

This patient is slightly hypertensive, but not enough to be worrisome in this setting. To eliminate other potentially serious cardiovascular issues, blood pressure reading should always be taken in both arms. When blood pressure measurement was repeated, the results were as follows: Left arm, 140/78 mmHg; right arm, 138/80 mmHg.

## Electrocardiogram (ECG)

The ECG shows no signs of ischemia, such as ST–T-wave abnormalities. Heart rate is regular, and the patient is in normal sinus rhythm. Luckily, an ECG readout from an earlier visit is available for comparison, and it looks similar.

When possible, it is always helpful to compare the ECG obtained during the current visit with any prior reading that you can obtain. Aside from any ischemic findings on ECG, it is important to rule out any signs of pericarditis or pulmonary embolism as those conditions can both present with chest pain and ECG changes. In this patient's case, his ECG is completely normal.

## Chest Radiograph

The chest film for this patient is normal. That means there are no signs of cardiomegaly, heart failure, or infection, or widened mediastinum that could be suggestive of aortic dissection. Remember, you are trying to determine if this patient's symptoms are the result of an acute cardiac problem. In order to do that, ruling out what the problem is not is just as important as determining what it is.

## Biomarkers and Lab Results

The initial troponin T level is undetectable. Older troponin assays to detect myocardial ischemia usually rise 6 to 12 hours after the episode of pain. Modern assays detect myocardial ischemia as early as 3 to 4 hours after onset of myocardial damage (Mangla & Gupta, 2015). The D-dimer level was also unremarkable.

This is another reason why questioning the patient about onset and duration of symptoms is important. As noted in the initial presentation, the patient came to the emergency department at 1900. His pain occurred at 11 a.m., so it has been more than 6 hours and the initial biomarker is negative. Regardless of whether older or more modern troponin assays are being used, a negative value in this setting should reassure the clinician that the patient has not had myocardial injury. These data would direct the clinician to consider a noncardiac cause of his symptoms as more likely than a cardiac cause.

The CBC and chemistry panel are unremarkable as well. A significant white blood cell count on the CBC should make the clinician think about a possible infectious component that might be related to his symptoms. In addition, any anemia or abnormal electrolyte values could also move the evaluation further away from a cardiac cause.

## Other Data

Other relevant data are available through review of his medication list. The first provider did not inquire about medications, but only assumed that what was noted in the chart was still up to date. The second provider asked specifically about his medication list and was able to identify a critical piece of information: the patient had stopped taking omeprazole 1 week earlier. In addition, the second provider also asked about ticagrelor and clopidogrel. These medications are P2Y12 inhibitors that are prescribed when patients undergo cardiac stent procedures. We know from the patient's history he had a stent implanted. The stent procedure took place 4 years ago, and the patient stated he took clopidogrel for 2 months and then was told he no longer needed it.

A cardiovascular clinician considering this information would likely assume that the type of stent implanted in this patient was a bare metal stent rather than a drug-eluting stent. According to the most recent American College of Cardiology/American Heart Association (ACC/AHA) guidelines, use of ticagrelor and clopidogrel is recommended for at least 1 month after placement of a bare metal stent and for at least 6 to 12 months after placement of a drug-eluting stent (Levine et al, 2016).

It is noted that the patient has a history of hypertension, hyperlipidemia, and type 2 diabetes. His other medications reflect management of those concurrent problems and are as follows: amlodipine, 5 mg daily; omeprazole, 20 mg daily (which the patient has not taken for the past week); simvastatin, 40 mg nightly; metformin, 500 mg twice daily; aspirin, 81 mg daily; and hydrochlorothiazide, 25 mg daily.

There is no available assessment of the patient's lipid status, but if a cardiac diagnosis is pursued, this information would need to be obtained to make sure the dose of lipid-lowering therapy is adequate. Although his blood pressure was slightly elevated on arrival, this can also be reassessed if the patient is admitted and optimized if needed.

The patient's social history was reviewed and is negative for tobacco, alcohol, or illicit drugs. His surgical history is unremarkable. His family history is significant for hypertension and hyperlipidemia in his mother, father, and sister. His social history is also reviewed.

## DIFFERENTIALS AND DIFFERENCES IN EXAM

When examining a patient with chest pain, it is important to thoroughly evaluate the chest and upper abdomen specifically by auscultation and palpation in addition to other elements of the exam. The cardiovascular clinician needs to ensure the pain is not reproducible with palpation or movement. In addition, any murmurs, adventitious breath sounds, bruits, or edema should be noted. Once the exam is complete, that along with the history and objective data is used to formulate a differential diagnosis list.

The cardiovascular clinician examines the patient. The findings are as follows:

*General appearance:* Slender, well-nourished, and well-developed African American male.

*Head and neck:* Head is normocephalic and atraumatic, without evidence of lesions or masses. Sclera are anicteric. Neck is soft and supple, without thyromegaly or lymphadenopathy.

*Cardiac exam:* No elevation of jugular venous pressure. No carotid bruits. No abdominal or femoral bruits. Carotid upstroke is brisk. Peripheral pulses are palpable and symmetric. Auscultation of the heart reveals a regular rate and rhythm. S1 and S2 present. No S3 or S4. No murmurs, rubs, heaves, or lifts. Chest wall is nontender to palpation.

*Lungs:* Clear breath sounds bilaterally with symmetric expansion.

*Abdomen:* Soft, nontender. Bowel sounds present in all four quadrants. No hepatosplenomegaly. No hepatojugular reflux.

*Extremities:* Warm and dry. No evidence of edema, clubbing, or cyanosis.

*Neurological:* Alert and oriented ×3. Cranial nerves are intact. Motor strength is symmetric in bilateral upper and lower extremities. Sensation is intact. No focal neurological deficits.

All key information and data have now been obtained. Based on history A, the presentation appeared to be more cardiovascular in nature, right? The most likely diagnosis in the differential might be unstable angina.

Based on what the provider obtained in history B, however, the details in the history alone should have steered you in a noncardiac direction. With the objective data and exam being normal, the most likely diagnosis is gastro esophageal reflux, or heartburn.

In any patient with chest pain, the cardiovascular clinician should immediately formulate a differential diagnosis list while simultaneously interviewing the patient. The list can be exhaustive, but with each piece of information gathered, the list should become smaller as things are eliminated.

Differential Diagnoses of Chest Pain

- Aortic dissection
- Cholecystitis
- Costochondritis
- GERD
- Heart failure

- Mediastinitis
- Musculoskeletal pain
- Myocardial infarction
- Peptic Ulcer
- Pericarditis

- Pleurisy
- Pneumonia
- Pulmonary embolus
- Unstable angina

GERD, gastroesophageal reflux disease.

# PULLING IT ALL TOGETHER

## Working Through the Differential

We can eliminate heart failure, pneumonia, pleurisy, costochondritis, and musculoskeletal pain right away.

- The patient's chest radiograph was without infection, pulmonary edema, or pleural effusion. He had no leukocytosis to suggest infection.

- His pain did not change with deep breathing or movements as is often seen with costochondritis, pleurisy, and musculoskeletal pain.

- Mediastinitis is also unlikely since we know the patient has not had any recent chest surgery or procedures that involve the chest or esophagus.

- The presentation of mediastinitis is quite different from that described for this patient, and usually the patient appears acutely ill often with evidence of sepsis.

- The chest wall was nontender and the patient did not have a fever on presentation or any signs of infection.

Aortic dissection is also less likely as well for these reasons:

- The patient did not have back pain, which is often typical of that presentation.

- His blood pressures were nearly symmetric.

- There was no evidence of a widened mediastinum on chest film.

A diagnosis of pericarditis is also unlikely:

- The classic symptoms are often similar to those seen with costochondritis and musculoskeletal pain. Chest pain that is caused by pericarditis is often positional as well, which his pain was not.
- In addition, there were no ECG changes suggestive of pericarditis such as PR depression or ST-segment elevation.
- There were no physical exam findings such as a pericardial friction rub to suggest this diagnosis.

Pulmonary embolus typically presents with shortness of breath and tachycardia. On occasion, there are ECG findings associated with this acute condition. Although it is still a possible diagnosis, pulmonary embolus is much less likely than other diagnoses because the patient denied feeling short of breath, his heart rate is normal, and his d-dimer level is normal.

Cholecystitis can mimic cardiac ischemia; however, typically nausea and vomiting are present, along with abdominal tenderness and often fever. There is a relationship to food, and pain often is present in the shoulder blade. This diagnosis can certainly be considered, but it is less likely to be the cause of this patient's symptoms owing to lack of abdominal tenderness. An abdominal ultrasound can quickly confirm or eliminate this diagnosis completely.

Peptic ulcers often have no symptoms, or more commonly cause stomach pain. The symptoms usually occur between meals or after certain types of foods, and can also include heartburn, nausea, and vomiting. Long-term use of nonsteroidal anti-inflammatory pain relievers is associated with peptic ulcers since these medications can break down the stomach lining. This diagnosis is certainly a possibility, but it can be confirmed only with laboratory tests and endoscopy. We cannot eliminate it completely yet.

So, we are left with unstable angina, myocardial infarction, and GERD as possibilities. Based on the ECG and biomarkers, we know the patient has not had a myocardial infarction.

Does the patient have unstable angina or GERD? An acute cardiovascular issue, or one that is not life threatening? Let us review the highlights of the history again:

- The patient's pain arose after eating on both occasions.
- He has not taken omeprazole, which was prescribed for his GERD symptoms, for 1 week.
- He admits that the pain is similar to his reflux symptoms.
- Similar symptoms were not present when he had a cardiac event in the past.

**Likely Diagnosis:** Exacerbation of GERD.

---

### WHAT'S NEXT?

- *The patient is placed back on omeprazole and discharged from the emergency department.*
- He follows up with his primary care physician within 1 week.
- He reports no further episodes of burning or chest discomfort.
- To be thorough, his physician orders a stress test, the results of which are normal.

---

## SUMMARIZING THE SCENARIO

In this clinical case, two separate histories were taken by two different providers. If we had relied only on the history taken by the first provider, this patient would likely have been admitted for treatment and would have undergone cardiac evaluation by stress testing or coronary angiography. The workup would likely have been unremarkable, but his symptoms would have persisted, delaying an accurate diagnosis.

As a cardiovascular clinician, the second provider was able to gain much more information simply by taking a detailed history. Without any other data, that history should have led to a diagnosis that the problem was not an acute cardiovascular issue, but rather one of reflux. The objective data that were gathered further supported this analysis.

Nonetheless, patients with unstable angina can present with heartburn as their chief complaint (McGraw, 2015). This patient is also diabetic, and diabetic individuals can have silent ischemia or even atypical presentations of acute coronary syndromes (Khafaji & Suwaidi, 2014). Although the patient underwent stress testing as an outpatient, it would not have been unreasonable to have completed the stress test before leaving the emergency department.

In Chapter 2, we look at another example of chest pain by way of a somewhat different interaction between a patient and healthcare providers.

# REFERENCES

Chan, S., Maurice, A., Davies, S., & Walters, D. (2014). The use of gastrointestinal cocktail for differentiating gastro-oesophageal reflux disease and acute coronary syndrome in the emergency setting: A systematic review. *Heart, Lung and Circulation, 23,* 913–923. doi:10.1016/j.hlc.2014.03.030

Chest pain. (2009). *Mosby's Medical Dictionary* (8th ed.). Retrieved from http://medical-dictionary.thefreedictionary.com/chest+pain

Giugliano, R., Cannon, C., & Braunwald, E. (2015). Non-ST elevation acute coronary syndromes. In D. L. Mann, D. P. Zipes, P. Libby, & R. O. Bonow, *Braunwald's heart disease: A textbook of cardiovascular medicine* (10th ed., pp. 1155–1181). Philadelphia, PA: Elsevier/Saunders.

Grailey, K., & Glasziou, P. (2012). Diagnostic accuracy of nitroglycerine as a test of treatment for cardiac chest pain: A systematic review. *Emergency Medicine Journal, 29,* 173–176. doi:10.1136/emj.2010.103994

Khafaji, H., & Suwaidi, J. (2014). A typical presentation of acute and chronic coronary artery disease in diabetics. *World Journal of Cardiology, 6*(8), 802–813. doi:10.4330/wjc.v6.i8.802

Mangla, A., & Gupta, A. (2015). Troponins. Retrieved from: http://emedicine.medscape.com/article/2073935-overview

McGraw, R. (2015). *Cardiology—interventional specialty review and study guide.* Orlando, FL: StatPearls.

Rui, P., Kang, K., & Albert, M. (2013). National Hospital Medical Care Survey: 2013 Emergency Department Summary Tables. Retrieved from: http://www.cdc.gov/nchs/data/ahcd/nhamcs_emergency/2013_ed_web_tables.pdf

# CHAPTER 2

# Chest Pain: Another Encounter

In the scenario that opens this chapter, we compare the history obtained by two providers a bit differently than in Chapter 1. In that scenario, the presentation for a patient with chest pain was described and then various features were extracted and discussed. In this chapter, we look at the initial interaction between each provider and the patient to demonstrate variations in how information is obtained, and then identify gaps in the data.

## CASE SCENARIO

Emergency medical services (EMS) arrive at the emergency department with a 52-year-old White male who awoke from sleep with chest pain. His initial blood pressure was 136/70 mmHg, pulse was 109 beats per minute, respiratory rate was 14 breaths per minute, oxygen saturation was 100% on room air, and he was afebrile. The emergency physician asks the patient the following questions to obtain a history:

Q: **Can you tell me what happened tonight to bring you to the emergency department?**

A: I had chest pain that woke me up.

Q: **What time did this occur?**

A: About midnight.

Q: **Can you tell me where the pain is located?**

A: Right here under my breastbone [patient points to his sternum].

Q: **What did you do when you first felt the pain?**

A: I got up, it seemed better, but not much, and then I took some TUMS thinking it was indigestion—but it didn't help.

Q: **Did the pain get better or worse with any movement or activity?**

A: No, I don't think so.

Q: **Did you have any other symptoms associated with the pain?**

A: No.

Q: **What level was your pain initially on a scale of 0 to 10 (0 being no pain, 10 being severe), and what is it now?**

A: It was a 10 but got better once the paramedics gave me aspirin. Now it's a 7 out of 10.

Q: **Do you have any history of heart disease?**

A: No.

Q: **Do you have any history of high blood pressure, high cholesterol, diabetes, or smoking?**

A: No.

The emergency physician obtains an ECG, which does not show any ischemia. Sublingual nitroglycerin is administered but does not improve the patient's symptoms. Initial vital signs are within normal limits except for mild tachycardia (heart rate of 110 beats per minute). Labs are drawn, which are notable only for a troponin T level of 0.09 ng/mL and a white blood cell (WBC) count of 11,000. The chest radiograph is also unremarkable. An exam is performed and is negative for any findings.

The emergency physician calls the on-call cardiovascular clinician at 0300 to evaluate this patient, who is believed to be having a non–ST-segment elevation myocardial infarction (NSTEMI). The emergency physician summarizes the information (history A) to the cardiovascular clinician.

# HISTORY A

*A 52-year-old White man with no prior cardiac history and no cardiac risk factors comes into the emergency department via EMS with complaints of substernal chest pain that awoke him from sleep around midnight. He thought the pain was indigestion and took TUMS, but it did not improve, so he called 911. He denies the pain being associated with movement. Initially, the pain was 10 out of 10 on a pain scale. Paramedics gave him 4 chewable baby aspirin, which gave him some relief, bringing the pain to 7 out of 10. He's received 1 sublingual nitroglycerin tablet in the emergency department with no further relief of pain. His exam was unremarkable. The initial ECG appears normal; however, his initial troponin T is 0.09 ng/mL. Basic chemistry panel and complete blood count (CBC) are otherwise normal except for a mildly elevated WBC count of 11,000. Chest radiograph is unremarkable for any acute process.*

Based on the preceding information, the cardiovascular clinician is already formulating a differential diagnosis. It sounds as though this patient could be having a NSTEMI, but in order to confirm this diagnosis, more information needs to be gathered, and quickly, to ensure timely treatment.

Before we examine how the next history is taken, are there any key features missing from the initial history taken by the emergency physician? Was that history detailed enough to lead you to the right diagnosis? Let us see what other questions the cardiovascular clinician asks to further evaluate the chief complaint.

Upon evaluating the patient, the following vital signs are obtained: Blood pressure, 138/72; pulse, 105 beats per minute; respiratory rate, 16 breaths per minute; oxygen saturation, 99% on room air; and the patient is afebrile. The cardiovascular clinician asks the patient the following questions:

Q: **What brings you to the emergency department?**

A: I had chest pain that woke me from sleep.

Q: **What time was that?**

A: Around midnight.

Q: Can you describe the pain for me? Is it sharp, burning, dull, or does it feel like a pressure or squeezing sensation? Have you had this pain before?

A: It was sharp at first, now it's dull. I've never felt anything like this.

Q: Where is it located?

A: Right here in the center of my chest. [The patient points to his sternum.]

Q: What is your level of pain now on a scale of 0 to10?

A: Around a 7.

Q: Do you notice the pain radiating to your back, jaw, neck, or arms?

A: No—it's staying right there.

Q: Are you short of breath, dizzy, nauseous, or sweaty with this pain or were you when it first occurred or did you feel an acid taste in your mouth or burning with it?

A: No, none of that.

Q: Have you been lightheaded with this pain or have you passed out from it?

A: No.

Q: I heard that you took TUMS to alleviate the pain. Did this help at all? How long did you wait before you took it?

A: I got out of bed and the pain was a little less sharp, but it didn't go away, so after 10 minutes or so I took some TUMS. It didn't help at all.

Q: The aspirin they gave you helped some, right, but not the nitroglycerin?

A: Yes, the aspirin did seem to take the edge off, but I didn't notice any change with the nitroglycerin.

Q: Does any movement make it better or worse; for example, moving your arms or sitting up versus lying down?

A: No. [He moves around in the bed.] I don't think so. I haven't tried lying down again since I woke up.

Q: I noticed you said the pain became less sharp when you got out of bed. Let me try something. (Currently the patient is lying at a 45-degree angle in the bed; the bed is adjusted to a supine position for a few minutes and then is lifted to a 90-degree angle.) Did you notice your pain changing at all as I repositioned you in the bed?

A: Yes—in fact I feel much better sitting up like this. The pain is less sharp.

Q: What is your pain level when you sit upright versus when you were lying flat?

A: It went back up to a 10 out of 10 lying down, but now it's about a 5 out of 10 sitting up.

Q: Do you feel the pain gets worse as you take a deep breath?

A: [Patient proceeds to take a deep breath and winces at end of inspiration.] Yes.

Q: Have you been sick recently, traveled recently, or been exposed to anyone who has been sick?

A: I haven't traveled anywhere, but I had the flu about a week ago.

Q: What were your symptoms at that time? Did you have cough, chest pain, or fever?

A: I had a cough, congestion, and fever, although I never checked it. But I had chills. I still feel really run down. No energy.

Q: Were you on any medication for your symptoms and do you take any medications on a daily basis?

A: I took some decongestant and Tylenol, but nothing else. I only take a daily multivitamin and fish oil capsules at night.

Q: Have you ever had a heart attack or stroke? Or do you have a history of high blood pressure, diabetes, or clots to your lungs or legs?

A: No.

Q: Do you exercise?

A: I cycle three times a week and lift weights twice a week.

Q: Have you done anything more strenuous than usual or feel that you have pulled any muscles?

A: No, I haven't worked out in 2 weeks because I was sick.

Q: Prior to tonight and even before your illness, have you felt more tired, had decreased endurance, or experienced any shortness of breath or chest pain?

A: No.

Q: Have you noticed any weight loss, weight gain, or changes in your bowel or bladder patterns?

A: No.

Q: Tell me about your day yesterday before going to bed last night. Did you do anything out of the ordinary or eat anything spicy or unusual for your diet?

A: No. I haven't had much of an appetite so I had some soup for dinner. I spent the whole day at home.

The patient's chief complaint has been thoroughly evaluated at this point. The cardiovascular clinician summarizes this information in history B.

# HISTORY B

*A 52-year-old White male with a recent history of presumed flu presents to the emergency department via EMS with complaints of substernal chest pain that awoke him from sleep around midnight. He has no past cardiac history or cardiac risk factors. His only symptom leading up to this episode was fatigue. He describes the pain as sharp, nonradiating, worse with deep breathing and lying down, and better with sitting upright and forward. He has not pulled any muscles recently or done any unusual activity or eaten anything out of the ordinary for his diet. The pain is not associated with shortness of breath, nausea or vomiting, syncope, near syncope, or diaphoresis. He attempted to alleviate the pain with TUMS; however, that was unsuccessful.*

*While in route to the emergency department he was treated with aspirin, which was somewhat effective in lessening the pain. Nitroglycerin did not give any further improvement and he currently states his pain is 5 out of 10 sitting upright.*

Utilizing *only* the history and no objective data, is a diagnosis of NSTEMI still at the top of your differential?

# KEY FEATURES OF THE HISTORY

The first history obtained (history A) seemed to be thorough, initially. It provided relevant and key information that was organized in a way that would likely lead any provider to a diagnosis of NSTEMI. Upon closer examination, however, the objective data, in conjunction with the history, are what essentially narrowed your thinking to this conclusion, right? Does that still hold true with history B? Did you need the objective data to change your differential diagnosis? Let us go back to the earlier question. What, if any, key features were missing from the initial history?

## Character

The character of the chest pain was identified in history A by asking the patient where the pain was located and the severity of pain. In history B, no questions were asked about what type of pain it was, or whether the pain radiated anywhere else.

In history B, the cardiovascular clinician asked detailed questions about whether the pain was a pressure, more of a dull ache, or was sharp. In addition, the patient was asked if the pain radiated to his neck, jaw, arms, or back. Every patient's perception of pain is different. It is important to identify the type of pain (sharp versus pressure) being experienced, particularly when talking about the chest as this symptom can drastically change the differential diagnosis.

## Timing and Duration

In both history A and history B, the patient was asked at what time of the day the pain occurred. The patient also disclosed what he was doing when it occurred. Pain that either awakens someone from sleep or occurs at rest can be a classic sign of an acute coronary syndrome or unstable angina, which makes this statement a key point of the patient's history (Giugliano, Cannon, & Braunwald, 2015). Duration was not directly asked, but it was clear that the patient was having ongoing pain without complete relief. In history B, the patient was asked if he had experienced this type of pain before. Addressing the frequency is an important point to establish for pain that might be consistent with a pattern of unstable angina.

## Associated Symptoms

Both providers asked the patient whether any other symptoms were associated with his pain. Although the answer was the same, how they asked the question was very different.

In history A, the patient was asked if he was having any other symptoms with his pain. In history B, the patient was asked whether he was feeling short of breath, nauseous, dizzy, sweaty, or had an acid taste in his mouth. These symptoms often occur in tandem with chest pain in situations of acute coronary syndromes and with other causes of chest pain, such as aortic dissection, gastroesophageal reflux disease (GERD), and pulmonary embolism, to name a few. The patient may not be able to identify that he had other symptoms if not prompted directly about those symptoms, which may have led to a false response when the provider in history A asked the question.

In addition, the provider in history B was thorough in asking the patient how he was feeling leading up to the event, including recent illnesses and exercise. In this line of questioning, the cardiovascular clinician was trying to determine whether the pain was associated with illness or caused by a pulled muscle. The fact that the patient had a recent history of viral illness is crucial in determining the right diagnosis, as you will soon see.

## Mitigating or Alleviating Factors

The provider in history A asked the patient what he did when he first felt the pain. He was asked a vague question about whether movement changed the pain, but was not asked specifically about what type of movement. This question yielded a false negative response from the patient. He gave away a key detail, though, that went unnoticed by the first provider, but was astutely caught by the second provider. The patient noted that when he stood, the pain was slightly better.

He relayed this observation in passing, though, and clearly did not recognize its importance. He took TUMS, which did not help to alleviate the pain, but the aspirin that the paramedics gave him did improve his pain to some degree.

When the second provider asked the patient if any movement made the pain better or worse, it was noted that the patient felt some difference upon standing and the provider questioned the patient about it. This information prompted the change in bed position to demonstrate this finding further. The patient was unaware of the connection until he was asked. In fact, putting the patient in an upright position was the only thing that improved his pain at all other than the aspirin. This was a critical piece of information that demonstrates the importance of paying close attention to everything the patient says. The patient was also asked whether deep breathing changed the pain, which it did. He again was unable to make this connection on his own without prompting from the provider. The positional nature of the pain as well as the relief with an anti-inflammatory should have definitely steered your thinking away from a diagnosis of NSTEMI.

# KEY FEATURES OF THE DATA

The key features of the data relevant to this patient's chief complaint are the vital signs, ECG, chest radiograph, and biomarkers and lab results. In addition, other data such as the medication list and relevant medical history need to be taken into consideration.

## Vital Signs

The following findings are reported at the time the cardiovascular clinician evaluates the patient:

*Blood pressure*: 138/70 mmHg

*Pulse*: 95 beats per minute

*Respirations*: 16 breaths per minute

*Oxygen saturation*: 99% on room air

*Temperature*: 37.0°C

A subsequent blood pressure reading is taken in each arm with the following results: right, 136/65 mmHg, left, 132/70 mmHg. This patient is slightly tachycardic, which can be a normal response in someone who is in pain. This finding is noteworthy as it can be indicative of pulmonary embolus as well as pericarditis.

## Electrocardiogram (ECG)

The ECG is read as sinus tachycardia without any acute abnormalities. The cardiovascular clinician carefully reviews the ECG and notes sinus tachycardia without any signs of ischemia such as ST-segment or T-wave abnormalities. There is depression of the PR segment in all leads. There is no prior ECG for comparison. The ECG is otherwise unremarkable.

## Chest Radiograph

The chest film does not demonstrate any findings of heart failure, pneumonia, or lung disease. The mediastinum is within normal limits and there is no cardiomegaly.

## Biomarkers and Lab Results

The initial troponin T level is abnormal at 0.09 ng/mL. As we learned with the case scenario in Chapter 1, modern troponin assays can rise as early as 3 to 4 hours after myocardial damage (Mangla & Gupta, 2015). This patient's pain awoke him from sleep around midnight and he is being evaluated in the emergency department around 3 a.m. His D-dimer level was checked and came back normal. His chemistry panel is within normal limits and shows no signs of kidney disease.

An abnormal troponin level in this setting should certainly narrow your focus to a cardiac cause for his symptoms. The CBC shows no signs of anemia and platelets are normal, but the patient's WBC is elevated at 11,000. Leukocytosis is frequently a sign of inflammation. It can also be due to a coronary event such as a NSTEMI (Scirica & Morrow, 2015) or other cardiac conditions such as pericarditis or myopericarditis (Doctor, Shah, Coplan, & Kronzon, 2016). We know that this patient had a recent viral illness, which may also contribute to the mildly abnormal WBC result.

## Other Data

The patient's medications are carefully reviewed with him and are notable only for a daily multivitamin and fish oil (1,000 mg) at night. He was taking over-the-counter cold and flu medicine during his viral illness. He is asked whether he had any history of cardiac disease, stroke, high blood pressure, diabetes, high cholesterol, or blood clots to his lungs or legs. Any risk factors associated with heart disease are relevant as is the absence of such. He has no past medical or surgical history other than left knee meniscus tear and repair about 10 years ago. He is an accountant and has no family history of coronary artery disease or any other cardiac problems. He does not smoke and drinks only on occasion. He denies any use of illicit drugs. He is seen by his primary care provider on a regular basis for routine physical examinations, but has never had a stress test or cardiac evaluation of any kind.

Assessing whether cardiac evaluation has occurred in the past can be helpful in deciding treatment and comparing data. Whenever patients state that they have no medical history, it is imperative that providers question them about the frequency of their primary care visits. If a patient has not been seen on a regular basis, he or she may harbor many underlying conditions that have yet to be detected. In this case, we can be reassured that the patient's medical history is up to date since he admits to seeing his primary care provider routinely.

# DIFFERENTIALS AND DIFFERENCES IN EXAM

At this point, the top differentials should be formulated based on the key findings of the data. The physical examination can often be the deciding factor when choosing the right diagnosis and a thorough examination of the chest, lungs, abdomen, and extremities is necessary. It should also focus on any physical findings that might confirm your diagnosis.

The cardiovascular clinician examines the patient. The findings are as follows:

*General appearance: Well-nourished, well-developed White male. Physically fit.*

*Head and neck: Head is normocephalic and atraumatic, without evidence of lesions or masses. Sclera are anicteric. Neck is soft and supple, without thyromegaly or lymphadenopathy.*

*Cardiac exam:* No elevation of jugular venous pressure. No carotid bruits. No abdominal or femoral bruits. Carotid upstroke is brisk. Peripheral pulses are palpable and symmetric. Auscultation of the heart reveals a regular rate and rhythm. S1 and S2 present. No S3 or S4. There is a pericardial friction rub best heard with the patient leaning forward. This is barely audible in the supine position. Chest wall is nontender to palpation.

*Lungs:* Clear breath sounds bilaterally with symmetric expansion. Pain noted on inspiration.

*Abdomen:* Soft, nontender. Bowel sounds present in all four quadrants. No hepatosplenomegaly. No hepatojugular reflux.

*Extremities:* Warm and dry. No evidence of edema, clubbing, or cyanosis.

*Neurological:* Alert and oriented ×3. Cranial nerves are intact. Motor strength is symmetric in bilateral upper and lower extremities. Sensation is intact. No focal neurological deficits.

Did the exam findings noted by the first provider correlate with those of the second provider?

The cardiovascular clinician heard a pericardial friction rub that was not heard by the first provider. Note that the rub was best heard with the patient sitting forward and was barely audible with the patient lying flat. It is quite possible the first provider did not listen to the patient in both positions, or there was too much background noise, or the rub simply was not present at that time. As this physical exam finding is not always present, it is important to listen for it in a patient with suspected pericarditis at regular intervals, with the patient in both sitting and supine positions (LeWinter & Hopkins, 2015). A presence of a pericardial friction rub is pathognomonic for pericarditis.

All key information and data have now been obtained. Based on history A, the presentation appeared to be cardiac in origin. With the abnormal troponin level, this finding further narrowed the diagnosis to NSTEMI. History B, which was obtained by the cardiovascular clinician, was much more elaborate and was based on the positional nature of the pain. Given these results, the working diagnosis of NSTEMI should have been replaced by that of acute pericarditis or myopericarditis. The objective data further supported this diagnosis.

Let's review the differential diagnoses for a chief complaint of chest pain, which we identified in Chapter 1, and discuss how the diagnosis of pericarditis was made in this case.

**Differential Diagnoses of Chest Pain**

- Aortic dissection
- Cholecystitis
- Costochondritis
- GERD
- Heart failure

- Mediastinitis
- Musculoskeletal pain
- Myocardial infarction
- Peptic ulcer
- Pericarditis

- Pleurisy
- Pneumonia
- Pulmonary embolus
- Unstable angina

GERD, gastroesophageal reflux disease

# PULLING IT ALL TOGETHER

## Working Through the Differential

We can eliminate heart failure, pneumonia, GERD, peptic ulcer, and cholecystitis.

- The patient's chest radiograph was without infection, pulmonary edema, or pleural effusion.
- Although he has a mildly elevated WBC count, his lungs were clear on exam, thus excluding a cause of pneumonia.
- A diagnosis of GERD is also less likely since there was no burning associated with his pain and TUMS did not alleviate the pain.
- Troponins are typically not elevated in the setting of GERD.
- There was no abdominal tenderness, nausea, or vomiting in relationship to food as seen with cholecystitis and often in the presence of a peptic ulcer.

Mediastinitis can be life threatening if not diagnosed in a timely manner.

- Often these patients appear acutely ill and may be septic.
- Although this patient is tachycardic with an elevated WBC, he does not meet the criteria for sepsis according to the Society of Critical Care Medicine and the European Society of Intensive Care Medicine (Singer et al., 2016).
- This patient does not have the other risk factors that are associated with this diagnosis.

Aortic dissection is a differential that needs to be ruled out quickly.

- The patient did not have any back pain that is often typical of this presentation.
- His pulses were symmetric and blood pressures taken on each arm were close in value.
- There was no evidence of a widened mediastinum on chest film.
- His pain did not radiate and it did change with movement.
- This diagnosis can be moved lower on the list.

Pulmonary embolus can be considered. Some of the characteristics of this pain fit with this diagnosis.

- The patient was tachycardic, but did not complain of any shortness of breath, which is often a key symptom of pulmonary embolus.
- ECG findings can suggest pulmonary embolus, but these findings were not evident in this case. However, the ECG can be completely normal with this diagnosis.
- He had no risk factors such as cancer, recent surgery, or travel.
- The D-dimer level is normal.
- Troponin levels can be slightly elevated in the presence of a pulmonary embolus.
- Although pulmonary embolus is not the most likely diagnosis, it cannot be completely eliminated yet.

What about the initial diagnosis of myocardial infarction or perhaps unstable angina? According to the joint European Society of Cardiology (ESC) and the American College of Cardiology, the classification of myocardial infarction includes the detection of a rise and fall of troponin with at least one of the following:

- Symptoms of ischemia
- Development of pathological Q waves in the ECG
- New or presumed new significant ST-segment and T-wave changes or new left bundle branch block (LBBB)
- Identification of an intracoronary thrombus by angiography or autopsy
- Evidence on imaging of new loss of viable myocardium or a new regional wall motion abnormality

This patient had a positive troponin value, but we have yet to develop a pattern that shows a rise and fall. His chest pain could be considered a symptom of ischemia if this is our diagnosis. It is difficult to distinguish unstable angina from a diagnosis of NSTEMI on initial presentation. However, the troponin value is what differentiates the two. In this case, given the abnormal troponin level, a diagnosis of unstable angina can be eliminated. Can we be so sure about NSTEMI?

So that leaves costochondritis, musculoskeletal pain, pleurisy, and pericarditis. All of these diagnoses have some similarities.

Costochondritis is inflammation of the cartilage that connects the rib to the breastbone. Typically, the chest wall is tender to palpation with this diagnosis. There is no evidence to suggest this is musculoskeletal pain. The patient was specifically asked about exercise and straining. Moving his arms around and stretching his chest did not change the pain as it would have if it were musculoskeletal in origin.

Pleurisy occurs when the lining around the lungs and chest cavity becomes inflamed. Often pleural effusions are seen on the chest film—a finding that this patient did not have. The pain with pleurisy can change with deep breathing and movement, but this is less likely to be the primary diagnosis in this patient.

Is it pericarditis then? In pericarditis, the pain typically worsens with lying down and deep breathing and improves with sitting up. The ECG can show PR depression or ST-segment elevation. A friction rub can be heard during auscultation but may be intermittent. In addition, troponin levels can be elevated. This patient was also tachycardic with a mild leukocytosis. Patients with pericarditis nearly always have an elevated WBC count and tachycardia (Doctor et al., 2016).

**Likely Diagnosis:** Pericarditis

Let us review the highlights of the history and data to see how this conclusion was reached:

- Pain worsened with deep breathing and supine positioning and improved with upright positioning.
- Anti-inflammatory medication improved the pain.
- The patient had a viral illness preceding his symptoms.
- A pericardial friction rub was heard on exam.
- ECG showed PR depression.

Most pericarditis cases in the United States are related to a viral infection. In developing countries, tuberculosis is a common cause (Imazio, Gaita, & LeWinter, 2015). According to the ESC guidelines, two out of the four following criteria must be present in order to diagnose acute pericarditis:

- Pericarditic chest pain
- Pericardial rub
- New widespread ST-elevation or PR depression on ECG
- Pericardial effusion

Acute pericarditis can be associated with myocardial involvement (myopericarditis) if there is an elevation in the biomarkers without evidence of left ventricular dysfunction (Adler et al., 2015). Viral illness is the most common cause of myopericarditis.

In this case scenario, the patient has three out of the four criteria to make a diagnosis of acute pericarditis. Furthermore, the elevated biomarkers suggest myocardial involvement. Acute pericarditis with associated myocardial involvement should be then referred to as myopericarditis according to the ESC guidelines.

WHAT'S NEXT?

- The patient is admitted to the hospital for further treatment.
- Subsequent troponin levels are drawn and are 0.09 ng/mL and 0.08 ng/mL. This pattern is not representative of the typical rise and fall seen with a diagnosis of NSTEMI; however, in cases of pericarditis with suspected myocardial involvement, it is not unreasonable to perform coronary angiography to rule out ischemia or significant coronary artery disease (Adler et al., 2015).

Correlation of symptoms and risk factors should be considered when making this decision. In this patient's case, coronary angiography is not pursued given the clinical presentation and low-risk profile.

- With a suspected diagnosis of pericarditis, an erythrocyte sedimentation rate (ESR) as well as a C-reactive protein (CRP) are drawn; both are elevated.
- An echocardiogram shows a normal ejection fraction of 62%, no wall motion abnormalities, no valvular abnormalities, and a tiny pericardial effusion.
- Cardiac magnetic resonance (CMR) is conducted, and the results are consistent with myopericarditis.
- No evidence for ischemia is found on CMR, and the ejection fraction is 59%.

Based on guideline-directed therapy, this patient is given high-dose aspirin and colchicine and started on a proton pump inhibitor for gastrointestinal prophylaxis. His pain resolves completely with a few doses of treatment. He is followed up in 1 month for repeat biomarker assays, which show inflammatory markers that have normalized. At that point, plans are initiated to taper the colchicine and aspirin over the course of the next few months.

# SUMMARIZING THE SCENARIO

This case scenario was similar to the scenario in Chapter 1 in that two separate histories were compared. The organization of the discussion of these two cases was slightly different in order to demonstrate the flow of the patient's interactions with each provider in a way that represents a typical encounter.

The key features of the history were identified in Chapter 1. The objective in this scenario was to realize immediately which features about the chief complaint were not given in the history obtained by the emergency physician. In responding to this case, you were required to identify the key features as you were reading the questions, rather than having them broken down for you, as was done in Chapter 1.

Once again, the history that each provider obtained led to a different diagnosis and a different treatment. The history that the cardiovascular clinician obtained was clearly more thorough and detailed. The questions that were asked may have seemed obvious and left you wondering how this information was not identified when the first provider interviewed the patient.

This case scenario is a great example of how providers often miss the bigger issue when a patient presents with what seems like a very straightforward complaint. The first provider probably felt that the complaint had been thoroughly evaluated. For example, associated movements and location of pain were questioned. However, the provider failed to be more specific about the effect of movement and positioning on the pain.

Once the cardiovascular clinician obtained this information, it should have been clear that the patient's pain was more consistent with pericarditis and not ischemia. The positive troponin value further led the emergency physician to focus only on the possibility of a NSTEMI rather than considering other factors that might also cause this value to be abnormal. The expertise of the cardiovascular clinician proved to be extremely beneficial in evaluating this patient.

## COMMON PITFALLS AND ASSUMPTIONS

Chest pain is a frequent complaint in the acute care setting. Patients typically seek medical attention because of the fear that they might be having a heart attack. In turn, providers often assume that this event is occurring to ensure that adequate workup and treatment is given in a timely manner, as this can be a life-threatening emergency.

Chest pain can be caused by many events or processes. Although patients may have a history of heart disease, chest pain does not always equate to ischemic pain in these individuals. Likewise, the absence of any cardiac history does not ensure that chest pain is not cardiac in nature.

It is common to assume that patients tell us everything about their complaint. Clinicians in a specialized role have a responsibility to dig deeper into the presenting complaint, background, and any associated factors as well as determine how the patient felt leading up to the presentation.

All of this information can be relevant, and many times patients are not able to make the connection on their own without the right questions to prompt them. Dissecting each key feature of a chief complaint helps the clinician formulate a diagnosis and a treatment plan much more efficiently, which ultimately leads the patient to resolution or improvement of symptoms and avoidance of unnecessary inpatient testing.

During the interview process, the process of determining the key features of character, timing and duration, associated symptoms, and mitigating or alleviating factors is often not broken down separately, as it was in Chapter 1. When taking a streamlined history, these features often overlap during questioning and are not necessarily obtained in that order. As in this case scenario, how and when the clinician elicits key information often depends on how much detail the patient gives on his or her own versus how much prompting is required. Many times, more questions arise based on what the patient communicates to the clinician. It is important that we think of these types of questions as we interview to make sure we obtain every possible detail related to the presenting symptom.

Breaking down the process allows us to examine more closely the techniques used in obtaining the history. The results are demonstrated in a clear and thorough documentation of the history of present illness in a way that summarizes the information and paints a clear picture of the patient's problem. This process is effectively illustrated in the histories summarized by the emergency physician and the cardiovascular clinician; however, the history obtained by the cardiovascular clinician included all necessary information in a succinct way in order to allow the reader to make a more accurate diagnosis.

# REFERENCES

Adler, Y., Charron, P., Imazio, M., Badano, L., Baron-Esquivias, G., Bogaert, J., . . . Tomkowski, W. (2015). 2015 ESC guidelines for the diagnosis and management of pericardial diseases. *European Heart Journal, 36*, 2921–2964. doi:10.1093/eurheartj/ehv318

Doctor, N., Shah, A., Coplan, N., & Kronzon, I. (2016). Acute pericarditis review. *Progress in Cardiovascular Disease, 59*(4), 349–359. doi:10.1016/j. pcad.2016.12.001

Giugliano, R., Cannon, C., & Braunwald, E. (2015). Non-ST elevation acute coronary syndromes. In D. L. Mann, D. P. Zipes, P. Libby, & R. O. Bonow, *Braunwald's heart disease: A textbook of cardiovascular medicine* (10th ed., 1155–1181). Philadelphia, PA: Elsevier/Saunders.

Imazio, M., Gaita, F., & LeWinter, M. (2015). Evaluation and treatment of pericarditis: A systemic review. *Journal of the American Medical Association, 314*(14), 1498–1506. doi:10.1001/jama.2015.12763

LeWinter, M., & Hopkins, W. (2015). Pericardial diseases. In D. L. Mann, D. P. Zipes, P. Libby, & R. O. Bonow, *Braunwald's heart disease: A textbook of cardiovascular medicine* (10th ed., pp. 1636–1657. Philadelphia, PA: Elsevier/ Saunders.

Mangla, A., & Gupta, A. (2015). Troponins. Retrieved from http://emedicine .medscape.com/article/2073935-overview

Scirica, B., & Morrow, D. (2015). ST-elevation myocardial infarction pathology, pathophysiology and clinical features. In D. L. Mann, D. P. Zipes, P. Libby, & R. O. Bonow, *Braunwald's heart disease: A textbook of cardiovascular medicine* (10th ed., pp. 1068–1094). Philadelphia, PA: Elsevier/Saunders.

Singer, M., Deutschman, C., Seymour, C., Shankar-Hari, M., Annane, D., Bauer, M., . . . Angus, D. (2016). The third international consensus definitions for sepsis and septic shock. *Journal of the American Medical Association, 315*(8), 801–810. doi:10.1001/jama.2016.0287

# CHAPTER 3

# Shortness of Breath: A First Look

## DEFINITION AND SIGNIFICANCE OF SHORTNESS OF BREATH

According to the *Gale Encyclopedia of Medicine* (2008), shortness of breath, or dyspnea, is defined as a "feeling of difficult or labored breathing that is out of proportion to the patient's level of physical activity." This can mean a variety of things to different patients. Many patients describe shortness of breath as a sensation of tightening in the chest, suffocation, air hunger, or breathlessness.

It was reported in the National Hospital Ambulatory Medical Care Survey that 3.4 million people presented to emergency departments in the United States in 2013 with complaints of shortness of breath (Rui, Kang, & Albert, 2013). Shortness of breath can be a symptom of a wide variety of disease processes and often these patients are in distress, making it difficult to obtain a comprehensive history. In addition, shortness of breath can arise when one illness is superimposed on another, making it an even greater challenge to diagnose and treat.

Cardiovascular clinicians are often asked to evaluate patients with this chief complaint as it can be a manifestation of heart failure, acute coronary syndrome, or other serious and acute cardiac conditions. The case scenarios presented in this chapter and in Chapter 4 are outlined in a similar fashion to those in Chapters 1 and 2. Once again variations in the history are demonstrated and reviewed as it relates to a chief complaint of shortness of breath.

## CASE SCENARIO

It is 3 p.m. and the cardiovascular clinician is called to evaluate a patient in the emergency department for possible heart failure. The initial history, labeled history A, was obtained by the emergency department provider. History B is taken by the consulting cardiovascular clinician. The consulting clinician is given the following information by the emergency department provider.

# HISTORY A

*A 59-year-old African American female with a past medical history of end-stage renal disease (ESRD)—thought to be secondary to hypertension, anemia, insulin-dependent type 2 diabetes mellitus, and hyperlipidemia—presents with complaints of shortness of breath for the past 10 days. She is in town visiting family and is due to start dialysis in 3 weeks in her hometown. Her nephrologist recently increased her dose of furosemide due to these complaints but she has not felt any improvement. She denies any edema more than her baseline and denies any chest pain or weight gain. She reports her symptoms are mainly worse when she is moving about, but lately feels short of breath sometimes at rest. She does not have a history of coronary artery disease (CAD) or heart failure. She is hypertensive here in the emergency department, but her exam is otherwise unremarkable.*

Available data thus far are as follows:

## VITAL SIGNS

*Blood pressure*: 160/95 mmHg

*Pulse*: 80 beats per minute

*Respirations*: 18 breaths per minute

*Oxygen saturation*: 98% on room air

*Temperature*: 36.7°C

(continued)

## VITAL SIGNS (*continued*)

### Biomarkers, Lab Results, and Diagnostic Tests

Troponin T is 0.14 ng/mL in the setting of creatinine of 4.6 mg/dL, BUN is 85 mg/dL, and glucose is 162 mg/dL. The rest of the chemistry panel is normal. The CBC is notable only for hemoglobin of 9.5 g/dL and hematocrit of 29%. The D-dimer test is unremarkable BNP is 220 pg/mL. A chest radiograph is clear of edema, effusions, or pneumonia. The ECG shows mild T-wave flattening in inferior leads but is otherwise normal.

### Home Medications

These are documented as follows: Sertraline, 50 mg daily; omeprazole, 20 mg daily; nifedipine, 30 mg daily; metoprolol, 50 mg twice daily; furosemide, 40 mg daily; folic acid daily; calcitriol daily; insulin 70/30 per sliding scale with meals; and atorvastatin, 40 mg every night.

Based on all the preceding information, do you think this clinical picture is one of heart failure?

The consulting cardiovascular clinician evaluates the patient and summarizes that information in history B.

# HISTORY B

*A 59-year-old African American female with a past medical history of ESRD secondary to hypertension, anemia, insulin-dependent type 2 diabetes mellitus, and hyperlipidemia presents to the emergency department with a 10-day history of progressive shortness of breath. She describes this as an inability to catch her breath. Her symptoms were gradual in onset are not associated with chest pain, diaphoresis, nausea, vomiting, lightheadedness, or syncope. She does note that she has had "tightness" in her chest on occasion when she is short of breath, but she relates this to rapid breathing during those moments.*

*She denies any palpitations and denies any fever, cough, recent illness, sick contacts, or travel. She initially noticed she had trouble catching her breath when climbing stairs and now she has shortness of breath with daily activities. She denies orthopnea or paroxysmal nocturnal dyspnea (PND), but does endorse some breathlessness at rest on occasion that has now been occurring for the past 2 days. She has felt more fatigued within this time frame as well. She denies any changes in her weight or any abdominal bloating. She has chronic ankle swelling that occurs at the end of the day, but this has not changed from baseline.*

*She is scheduled to start dialysis in her hometown in 3 weeks and was evaluated by her nephrologist for these complaints within the past week. At that time her dose of furosemide (20 mg) was increased to 40 mg daily. She has had no improvement in her symptoms. She denies any changes to her urinary frequency, pattern, or consistency. She reports her systolic blood pressures have been in the 140 to 150 mmHg range at home and that this is her baseline. She denies any recent dietary indiscretions such as increased salt or fluid intake and has been compliant with her prescribed medications. She denies having any history of heart failure or CAD. Her cardiovascular risk factors include a positive family history, hypertension, hyperlipidemia, diabetes, and a remote smoking history. She has never had a stress test or any cardiovascular testing aside from an ECG.*

Does this history paint a different picture? Does this patient have heart failure?

## KEY FEATURES OF THE HISTORY

Each history includes all of the information gathered from each provider at the time they evaluated the patient. Once again, history B is more detailed and perhaps led your differential diagnosis in another direction. We discuss the exam and other objective data obtained by the cardiovascular clinician later in this section, but for now let us again compare those key features of the chief complaint to identify differences in questioning that led to each history. Remember, those features are character (including location and severity), timing (including onset) and duration, associated symptoms, and any mitigating or alleviating factors.

## Character

The provider in history A identified the character of the chief complaint by asking the patient the following questions:

Q: **Why did you come to the emergency department today?**

A: I have been having shortness of breath.

Q: **Are you short of breath all the time or only with certain activities?**

A: Mostly with activity, but I have been short of breath doing nothing at times as well.

Q: **Have you ever had these symptoms before?**

A: No.


Here is how the provider in history B questioned the patient about the character:

Q: **What brought you here to the emergency department today?**

A: I have been having shortness of breath.

Q: **Have you ever experienced these symptoms before?**

A: No.

Q: **Describe the shortness of breath to me. Do you feel like it is hard to breathe or is it hard to catch your breath?**

A: I feel like I can't catch my breath sometimes.

Q: **Are you short of breath mainly with activity or do you have these symptoms at rest as well?**

A: Mostly with activity, but lately I have had them at rest too.


With a chief complaint of shortness of breath, there is not a lot more about character that can be asked. The cardiovascular clinician asked about whether the patient had a sense of breathlessness, or an inability to breathe. These differences are subtle, but worth noting. With chest pain, the character can be one of the most important things to define, but with a complaint of shortness of breath, timing, duration, and associated factors are more relevant.

## Timing and Duration

The provider in history A asked the following questions associated with the timing and duration of symptoms:

Q: **How long have you had these symptoms?**

A: For about 10 days.

Q: **Have they gotten worse, better, or stayed the same during that time?**

A: Initially I only felt short of breath with activity, but lately I feel it at rest, too, so I would say it's getting worse.

Here is what the provider in history B asked to illicit details about timing and duration of symptoms:

Q: **How long have you had these symptoms?**

A: For about 10 days.

Q: **Did the shortness of breath come on suddenly one day, or were the symptoms more gradual?**

A: Gradual. I can't recall a certain time specifically that I noticed it.

Q: **Do you know what you were doing when you began to notice you were short of breath?**

A: I noticed when I climbed my stairs that I couldn't get my breath, which is not normal for me. I started to get short of breath just getting dressed and showering, too.

Q: **When did you start to notice you were having shortness of breath at rest?**

A: About 2 days ago.

Q: **Do you have shortness of breath that awakens you from sleep, or do you have difficulty lying flat without getting short of breath?**

A: No. I have not had any of that.

Both providers asked questions about timing and duration. The emergency department provider asked whether the patient's symptoms had changed but did not ask for details about the specific timing in which her symptoms worsened.

The cardiovascular clinician, however, asked questions that elicited a pattern of progression by asking when the patient began to have symptoms at rest. Does this subtle detail drastically change the diagnosis? Perhaps not, but establishing a timeline can help narrow the differential diagnosis as it relates to the treatment received or any other associated symptoms.

The cardiovascular clinician also asked about orthopnea and PND, which can be key features in heart failure exacerbations and are important to determine in any patient with shortness of breath who you suspect may have heart failure.

## Associated Symptoms

The first provider asked the following questions about associated symptoms:

Q: **Have you had any chest pain with the shortness of breath?**

A: No.

Q: **Have you experienced any weight gain or swelling in your ankles?**

A: My weight hasn't changed. My ankles always swell a bit, but they don't seem any worse than normal.

The second provider asked the following questions about associated symptoms:

Q: **Have you had any chest pain, chest tightness, burning, or aching with your shortness of breath?**

A: No chest pain. I do have some tightness across my chest when I'm really struggling to catch my breath. I assume it's related to that.

Q: **Have you had any swelling in your legs, abdominal fullness, or weight gain or loss?**

A: My ankles always swell a bit at the end of the day but no worse than normal. I haven't noticed any changes in weight or abdominal bloating.

Q: **Have you been sick recently? Around anyone who is sick or had any cough or fever with this?**

A: No cough or fever. No one has been sick around me.

Q: **Do you have any sensation that your heart is racing, or do you have any palpitations?**

A: No.

Q: **Have you had any nausea, vomiting, sweats, dizziness, or have you passed out with these symptoms?**

A: None of that.

Q: **Have you noticed any increased fatigue or weakness?**

A: Yes, actually. I've been really tired—more so in the past 2 days.

Q: **Have you had any changes to your diet? Increased fluid or salt intake more than normal?**

A: No. I hardly eat any salt and I drink about the same amount of fluid every day.

The cardiovascular clinician asked many more details about associated symptoms than the emergency department provider. Notice how both asked about chest pain, but the cardiovascular clinician asked about tightness, aching, and burning. This patient did not associate chest pain with the tightness that she was feeling, which is why she likely answered "no" when asked by the first provider. In health care we use the term "chest pain" to encompass any chest syndrome of pain, squeezing, tightness, and so forth. Many patients do not understand this and view each symptom separately, which demonstrates the need to be specific.

In addition, both providers asked about weight gain and swelling, which are often symptoms of heart failure. The second provider went on to ask about abdominal bloating, which can also be a sign of heart failure. The patient was questioned about symptoms that can contribute to shortness of breath with other conditions, such as palpitations, dizziness, and syncope, which may signify an arrhythmia, as well as symptoms that might suggest a respiratory infection, such as fever, cough, and sick contacts, and finally symptoms that can be associated with ischemia: fatigue, nausea, and vomiting. These questions help readily eliminate other causes or narrow the focus to a specific diagnosis or plan. Asking about dietary indiscretion is also important when evaluating a patient for heart failure since many of these patient types have exacerbations due to increased salt or fluid intake.

## Mitigating or Alleviating Factors

The provider in history A asked the following question about mitigating and alleviating factors:

Q: **Have you seen your doctor or taken anything to improve these symptoms?**

A: I went to my nephrologist about 5 days ago and he increased my Lasix (furosemide) to 40 mg a day from 20 mg daily, but it did not help.

The provider in history B asked the following questions:

Q: **Have you done anything about these symptoms before today— changed medications or seen your doctor?**

A: I went to my nephrologist about 5 days ago and he increased my Lasix to 40 mg daily from 20 mg. I have not noticed any improvement.

Q: **Did you notice any change in your urinary output or frequency or pattern once the Lasix was increased?**

A: I don't think so. I don't urinate often anyway and I'm due to start dialysis soon.

The earlier line of questioning about timing was able to extract other things about mitigating and alleviating factors as well. Both clinicians were able to identify that the shortness of breath was worse initially with activity and now it sometimes occurs at rest.

Although asking about urinary frequency and output does not directly relate to mitigating or alleviating factors, the clinician's question was in direct response to a change in the patient's diuretic dosage and assessing that response is important to document, particularly in the setting of heart failure. Diuresis is the mainstay of heart failure management, so the absence of any increased diuresis with the increased dose of furosemide is worth highlighting. However, keep in mind that with ESRD, diuretics often become less effective (Rosenberg, 2016). In this patient, no variables other than activity and rest influenced the complaint of shortness of breath.

# KEY FEATURES OF THE DATA

The key features of the data include all of the laboratory and imaging data available as well as medications and relevant past medical, surgical, social, and family histories. With a chief complaint of shortness of breath, the key objective features are as follows: Vital signs, ECG, chest radiograph, biomarkers, BNP, basic chemistry panel, and CBC. These data were available at the time the emergency department provider contacted the cardiovascular clinician for consultation. Let us discuss the data further.

## Vital Signs

The following findings were reported:

*Blood pressure*: 160/95 mmHg

*Pulse*: 80 beats per minute

*Respirations*: 18 breaths per minute

*Oxygen saturation*: 98% on room air

*Temperature*: 36.7°C

This patient is hypertensive. She did indicate that her baseline systolic blood pressure was slightly lower at 140 to 150 mmHg. We know she has a history of hypertension likely leading to her ESRD. Blood pressures were repeated in each arm by the cardiovascular clinician and were as follows: Left, 158/82 mmHg; right, 156/82 mmHg. Continued management of her blood pressure and additional therapies need to be considered in her treatment plan. Her respiratory rate is at the upper limits of normal, but she is not tachypneic.

## Electrocardiogram (ECG)

Her ECG demonstrates T-wave flattening in the inferior leads (II, III, aVF). We have no other ECG to which to compare this finding; it can be non-specific, a sign of ischemia, or the patient's baseline. Serial ECGs would help the clinician define this pattern and look for changes. Obtaining a prior ECG from her primary physician would also prove useful. No arrhythmias were noted, and there were no overt signs of ischemia such as ST depression or elevation, or T-wave inversion. There are no changes consistent with pericarditis or pulmonary embolus and no evidence of conduction abnormalities.

## Chest Radiograph

The chest film is one of the most important pieces of data when evaluating a patient with shortness of breath. As a clinician, you should be looking for signs of pulmonary edema, effusions, evidence of infection or lung disease, and heart size. This patient's film was absent any of those findings and her heart size was normal.

## Biomarkers and Lab Results

The troponin T value was 0.14 ng/mL. It is well known that patients with chronic kidney disease can have elevated troponin levels. Even in the era of high sensitivity troponins, diagnosing acute coronary syndromes in this population can be challenging. The other data as well as serial changes of the troponin levels are more sensitive for a diagnosis of acute myocardial infarction among patients with chronic kidney disease (Parikh, Seliger, & deFilippi, 2015).

In addition, troponins are considered much more specific for myocardial injury than the cardiac marker creatinine kinase myocardial b fraction (CKMB), and should always be used when available. Elevation in both troponin I and CKMB is possible in patients with chronic kidney disease and cannot predict the presence of ischemia in isolation among this group (Kiranmayi, Lakshmi, Tagore, & Kambar, 2015). In addition, troponin levels can also be detected in the setting of heart failure and have been studied as a prognostic indicator for mortality and adverse cardiovascular outcomes (Grodin & Tang, 2013). The significance of an isolated troponin value in this patient's case is unclear. It should prompt you to obtain serial levels to assess for change.

The creatinine and BUN are abnormal as expected in the setting of ESRD. The patient's baseline creatinine is initially unclear.

The cardiovascular clinician did inquire about her normal creatinine level and the patient stated it was around 4 mg/dL. There were no other abnormalities in the basic chemistry panel. Her CBC shows no elevation in her WBC count to indicate infection. She has a mild anemia likely related to her chronic kidney disease which correlates with her history. A D-dimer test, obtained to evaluate for the possibility of a pulmonary embolus as a cause for her symptoms, was also negative.

The BNP is slightly elevated at 220 pg/mL. It is well known that BNP levels are elevated in patients in conditions of increased volume or pressure states as in heart failure (Kim & Januzzi, 2011). The use of BNP is most helpful when diagnosing heart failure in the acute care setting, especially if the diagnosis is unclear. Elevated BNP levels have also been found in patients with other conditions, such as acute and chronic renal insufficiency, pulmonary diseases, and cardiac causes, to name a few (Mangla, 2014). In addition, elevated BNP levels have been associated with the presence and severity of coronary artery disease in patients with unstable angina and non–ST-segment elevation myocardial infarction (NSTEMI; Romel et al., 2014). The elevated level of BNP in this patient does not necessarily help us diagnose heart failure or cardiac ischemia given her comorbid condition of ESRD, but it may be useful in determining further diagnostic evaluation.

## Other Data

Medications usage was carefully obtained from the patient and documented in the chart by the first provider. These agents were again verified by the second provider. The patient is compliant, and the listed dosages are accurate. She had taken all her morning medications before coming to the emergency department. Her past medical history is notable for the ESRD with plans to start hemodialysis in a few weeks in her hometown. She is scheduled to have dialysis access placed a few days beforehand.

She has been told her renal disease is likely secondary to longstanding high blood pressure. She also has type 2 insulin-dependent diabetes mellitus which is managed with sliding scale insulin. She has hyperlipidemia but is unsure of when her cholesterol was last checked. She sees her nephrologist on a regular basis. Her family history is positive for hypertension and coronary artery disease in her father (diagnosed at the age of 60); he is now deceased. Her mother and brother have hypertension, as well. She has a remote smoking history of 1 pack per day for 25 years. She quit at the age of 50. She denies any alcohol use or abuse and does not use any illicit drugs. Her medications reflect management of these ongoing medical issues.

## DIFFERENTIALS AND DIFFERENCES IN EXAM

The examination of a patient with shortness of breath is similar to that of any patient with a suspected cardiac diagnosis. All providers develop a pattern and a consistency to their exams regardless of the presenting symptoms; however, the cardiovascular clinician should focus on the subtle variations in the exam that call for their expertise. These findings may be missed by other clinicians. Inspection of the patient's appearance along with a careful evaluation of the chest, lungs, extremities, and vasculature should be the focus.

The cardiovascular clinician examines the patient and notes the following findings:

*General appearance*: Well-nourished, well-developed African American female in no acute distress.

*Head and neck*: Head is normocephalic and atraumatic, without evidence of lesions or masses. Sclera are anicteric. Neck is soft and supple, without thyromegaly or lymphadenopathy.

*Cardiac exam*: No elevation of jugular venous pressure (JVP). No carotid bruits. No abdominal or femoral bruits. Carotid upstrokes are brisk. Peripheral pulses are palpable and symmetric. Auscultation of the heart reveals a regular rate and rhythm. S1 and S2 present. No S3 or S4. No murmurs, rubs, heaves, or lifts. Chest wall is nontender to palpation.

*Lungs*: Clear breath sounds throughout all lung fields with symmetric expansion. Dyspnea noted intermittently during speech.

*Abdomen: Soft, nontender. Bowel sounds present in all four quadrants. No hepatosplenomegaly. No hepatojugular reflux.*

*Extremities: Warm, dry. Trace bilateral ankle edema. No clubbing or cyanosis.*

*Neurological: Alert and oriented ×3. Cranial nerves are intact. Motor strength is symmetric in bilateral upper and lower extremities. Sensation is intact. No focal neurological deficits.*

Now that all the key information and data have been obtained, what do you think is the most likely diagnosis? Do you agree with the emergency department provider that this is a presentation of heart failure? Did the cardiovascular clinician's evaluation confirm this diagnosis or did it lead you in another direction?

The differential diagnosis list for shortness of breath is extensive. Many chronic conditions can cause shortness of breath, but based on this scenario we can focus on those representative of an acute issue.

### Differential Diagnoses of Shortness of Breath

- Anaphylaxis
- Cardiac tamponade
- COPD/asthma exacerbation
- Heart failure
- Interstitial lung disease
- Lung cancer
- Myocardial infarction
- PAH
- Pneumonia/respiratory infection
- Pneumothorax
- Pulmonary embolus
- Unstable angina

COPD, chronic obstructive pulmonary disease; PAH, pulmonary arterial hypertension

This case scenario presents a challenging dilemma. The cardiovascular clinician was able to obtain more details about the chief complaint, but the diagnosis is not yet clear. What were the differences between the two providers that may have changed the primary working diagnosis from heart failure to something else? Let us review the highlights:

| Emergency Department Provider (History A) | Cardiovascular Clinician (History B) |
|---|---|
| • Shortness of breath 10 days | • Shortness of breath 10 days |
| • Occurs at rest | • Some chest tightness and fatigue |
| • No edema or weight gain | • Occurring at rest over past 2 days |
| • Exam normal | • No weight gain, PND, abdominal bloating, edema, orthopnea |
| • Chest film clear | • Exam not consistent with heart failure |
| • BNP and troponin abnormal | • BNP and troponin abnormal |
| • No improvement with furosemide | • ESRD initiating dialysis soon |
| • ESRD initiating dialysis soon | • ECG with T-wave flattening inferiorly |
| • ECG without ischemic findings | • Multiple risk factors for CAD |

PND, paroxysmal nocturnal dyspnea; BNP, brain natriuretic peptide; ESRD, end-stage renal disease; ECG, electrocardiogram; CAD, coronary artery disease

# PULLING IT ALL TOGETHER

## Working Through the Differential

What diagnoses on this list can we eliminate right away? How about ana-phylaxis? This patient is clearly not having an allergic reaction based on her evaluation. We can also eliminate pneumonia and any respiratory infection.

- She does not have an elevated white count.
- Her chest film is negative for an infectious process.
- She denies any cough associated with her symptoms.

It is possible to have a false-negative chest film in patients with pneu-monia (Maughan, Asselin, Carey, Sucov, & Valente, 2014); however, her exam findings do not support this diagnosis.

Pneumothorax would have been present on chest film. Breath sounds were clear on exam, so this diagnosis can easily be eliminated as well.

This patient has a remote smoking history, but no documented diagnosis of chronic obstructive pulmonary disease (COPD) or asthma. She has no wheezing present on exam and chest film does not demonstrate a barrel chest appearance on the lateral view that is sometimes seen with COPD. There are no changes suggestive of emphysema either such as flattened hemidiaphragm or hyperinflation. Most of the time COPD and asthma exacerbations are triggered by a bacterial or viral infection (Kurai, Saraya, Ishii, & Takizawa, 2013). She has had no preceding illness and no evidence of current infection, so we can eliminate this from our differential list as well.

Cardiac tamponade is considered a life-threatening emergency and requires urgent detection and treatment. Typical findings, such as elevated JVP, tachycardia, hypotension, and muffled heart sounds, are not present in this patient. An echocardiogram or a CT scan of the chest would completely eliminate this diagnosis, but based on her clinical exam we can put it near the bottom of our list.

The chest film did not show any evidence of interstitial lung disease or any nodules that may be suspicious for malignancy. Her history of tobacco use certainly puts her at increased risk for lung cancer. This diagnosis can still be considered, but only if all others have been ruled out. It is still not the most likely cause of her symptoms, but it should not be completely eliminated yet.

Pulmonary arterial hypertension (PAH) can be idiopathic or secondary to other conditions and it can cause enlargement of the right ventricle and pulmonary arteries, which can be seen on chest film. This patient did not have these findings. An echocardiogram would also be able to confirm this diagnosis. Based on the nature of her symptoms, it is less likely to be the cause, but we cannot completely eliminate it just yet.

Pulmonary embolus is a reasonable thing to consider in this patient. Her shortness of breath and episodic chest tightness are typical of this diagnosis. This was the rationale for performing a D-dimer test, which was negative. This finding can reassure us that she does not have a pulmonary embolus. D-Dimer tests produce very few false negatives and tend to have more levels of false positive results, which require imaging to completely rule out this diagnosis (Crawford et al., 2016).

So, we are left with heart failure, myocardial infarction, and unstable angina.

Heart failure is prevalent among patients with chronic kidney disease and ESRD (Segall, Nistor, & Covic, 2014). However, certain criteria must be present in order to make a diagnosis of heart failure. The Framingham criteria for diagnosing heart failure require the presence of two major criteria or one major and two minor criteria (Dumitru, 2016). Major and minor criteria are as follows:

| Major | Minor |
|---|---|
| Paroxysmal nocturnal dyspnea | Bilateral ankle edema |
| Neck vein distention | Nocturnal cough |
| Rales | Dyspnea on ordinary exertion |
| Cardiomegaly on chest film | Hepatomegaly |
| Acute pulmonary edema | Pleural effusion |
| S3 gallop | Decrease in vital capacity by one-third from maximum recorded |
| Increased central venous pressure | |
| (>16 cm $H_2O$ at right atrium) | Tachycardia |
| Hepatojugular reflux | |
| Weight loss (>4.5 kg in 5 days) in response to treatment | |

This patient demonstrates no major criteria and only minor criteria of dyspnea on ordinary exertion and perhaps bilateral ankle edema—although patient has longstanding baseline of mild ankle edema. She does not meet the criteria for heart failure based on this definition.

According to the European Society of Cardiology (ESC), there are now three types of heart failure: heart failure with reduced ejection fraction of less than 40% (HFrEF), heart failure with mid-range ejection fraction of 40% to 49% (HFmEF), and heart failure with preserved ejection fraction of 50% or greater (HFpEF; Ponikowski, et al., 2016). Without an echocardiogram, we do not know what this patient's ejection fraction is but according to the ESC guidelines, if her ejection fraction is reduced, symptoms and/or signs need only be present to make the diagnosis of heart failure. If her ejection fraction is midrange or preserved, increased levels of BNP need to be present as well as relevant structural heart disease or diastolic dysfunction along with symptoms and/or signs.

She has elevated BNP levels, which as discussed can be elevated in both ESRD and cardiac ischemia. We might be able to presume she has diastolic dysfunction due to her longstanding history of hypertension; however, without an echocardiogram we cannot confirm this. Her only symptom of heart failure is shortness of breath. She has no other symptoms, signs, or clinical exam findings to support this diagnosis.

It has been well documented that patients with chronic kidney disease have a high prevalence of coronary artery disease as do patients with diabetes. This patient has both conditions but has not yet been diagnosed with cardiovascular disease.

The cardiovascular clinician identified that the patient was experiencing chest tightness and fatigue along with her shortness of breath. This should have been the piece of information that turned your focus to a potential ischemic source of her symptoms rather than heart failure. The objective data of elevated BNP and troponin corroborate either diagnosis, but as mentioned previously, are not as helpful in the setting of ESRD. In Chapter 2 we identified the difference between unstable angina and a myocardial infarction or NSTEMI as a positive troponin value. This patient's troponin value may be chronically elevated, so we cannot determine whether she is having NSTEMI or unstable angina just yet. Remember, in these cases it is the pattern of the troponin levels and the serial changes that differentiate between unstable angina and NSTEMI (Parikh, Seliger, & deFilippi, 2015).

In general, women with coronary artery disease often present with atypical symptoms such as shortness of breath and fatigue rather than classic chest pain (Canto, Canto, & Goldberg, 2014). Furthermore, diabetic patients are also known to experience silent myocardial ischemia and infarction, often presenting with few or no symptoms at all

(Khafaji & Suwaidi, 2014). This patient is female, diabetic, and has ESRD, making it nearly impossible to make a diagnosis of myocardial infarction based on the data we have so far.

The history and data in isolation were not quite enough in this case scenario to make a definitive diagnosis. However, we were able to eliminate several diagnoses.

The comprehensive history taken by the cardiovascular clinician provided further insight into the chief complaint, which should have led us to think of ischemia as the cause of her symptoms and not heart failure. She has multiple risk factors for coronary artery disease, including a positive family history, positive tobacco history, hypertension, hyperlipidemia, and diabetes. In addition, she had progressive shortness of breath with chest tightness. She has no clinical findings of volume overload, no edema, no PND, and she had no improvement with furosemide.

**Likely Diagnosis:** NSTEMI

---

## WHAT'S NEXT?

- *The patient is admitted to the hospital.*
- She is not given further diuresis as there is no evidence of volume overload.
- A heparin drip is begun based on the hospital's acute coronary syndrome protocol.
- Serial troponin levels are drawn and are as follows: 0. 20 ng/mL, 0.18 ng/mL, 0.13 ng/mL. Once the second troponin level is obtained she is given ticagrelor, 180 mg, based on guideline-directed therapy for treatment of NSTEMI (Amsterdam et al., 2014). (Remember, her initial troponin level was 0.14 ng/mL, so the rise-and-fall pattern confirmed our diagnosis).
- She is scheduled for an echocardiogram, which demonstrates an ejection fraction of 64%, grade II diastolic dysfunction, and no significant valvular abnormalities. She has normal right ventricular size and function.
- She undergoes coronary angiography and is found to have severe multivessel disease; she is then referred for coronary artery bypass grafting.

---

## SUMMARIZING THE SCENARIO

This clinical case proved to be somewhat more of a challenge and demonstrated how normally reliable data can become unreliable with certain underlying conditions. Once again two providers presented histories based on the information they obtained from the patient.

The emergency department provider felt that the symptoms were consistent with heart failure. The detailed history obtained by the cardiovascular clinician was able to clarify that the symptoms were more consistent with ischemia than heart failure. Although this patient did not present with classic symptoms of chest pain, she did have chest tightness, progressive shortness of breath, and fatigue, which are features associated with cardiac ischemia—particularly in women and in diabetic patients. The expertise of the cardiovascular clinician enabled this information to be elucidated and synthesized in a way that supported this clinical picture.

The objective data always help solidify or negate any working diagnosis we have, but in this case initial data did not necessarily support the diagnosis of either the emergency department provider or the cardiovascular clinician. However, subsequent data, and the information gathered by the cardiovascular clinician, were enough to pursue an ischemic evaluation that let to prompt and timely treatment of this patient's NSTEMI.

If a heart failure diagnosis had been pursued, this patient would likely have received intravenous diuretics that would not have been effective; would not have received heparin; and would ultimately have suffered a delay in diagnosing the acute cardiac issue that led her to seek treatment.

In Chapter 4, we consider another example of shortness of breath by way of a somewhat different interaction between a patient and healthcare providers.

## REFERENCES

Amsterdam, E., Wenger, N., Brindis, R., Casey, D., Ganiats, T., Holmes, D., ... Zieman, S. (2014). AHA/ACC Guideline for the management of patients with non-ST-elevation acute coronary syndromes: A report of the American College of Cardiology/American Heart Association Task Force on Practice Guidelines. *Circulation, 135*(8), e344–e426. doi:10.1161/CIR.0000000000000134

Canto, J., Canto, E., & Goldberg, R. (2014). Time to standardize and broaden the criteria of acute coronary syndrome symptom presentations in women. *Canadian Journal of Cardiology, 30*, 721–728.

Crawford, F., Andras, A., Welch, K., Sheares, K., Keeling, D., & Chappell, F. (2016). D-dimer test for excluding the diagnosis of pulmonary embolism in hospital outpatient and accident and emergency populations. *Cochrane Database of Systematic Reviews, 8*. Article No. CD010864. doi:10.1002/14651858. CD010864.pub2

Dumitru, I. (2016). Heart failure. In H. H. Ooi (Ed.), *Medscape*. Retrieved from http://emedicine.medscape.com/article/163062-overview

Gale Encyclopedia of Medicine. (2008). Shortness of Breath. Retrieved from http://medical-dictionary.thefreedictionary.com/Shortness+of+Breath

Grodin, J., & Tang, W. (2013). Prognostic role of cardiac troponin in heart failure. Retrieved from http://www.acc.org/latest-in-cardiology/articles/2014/07/18/14/52/prognostic-role-of-cardiac-troponin-in-heart-failure

Khafaji, H., & Suwaidi, J. (2014). Atypical presentation of acute and chronic coronary artery disease in diabetics. *World Journal of Cardiology, 6*(8), 802–813. doi:10.4330/wjc.v6.i8.802

Kim, H., & Januzzi, J. (2011). Natriuretic peptide testing in heart failure. *Circulation, 123*(18), 2015–2019. doi:10.1161/CIRCULATIONAHA.110.979500

Kiranmayi, B., Lakshmi, A., Tagore, R., & Kambar, C. (2015). Evaluation of cardiac markers in chronic renal failure. *Journal of Dental and Medical Sciences, 14*(1), 46–52.

Kurai, D., Saraya, T., Ishii, H., & Takizawa, H. (2013). Virus-induced exacerbations in asthma and COPD. *Frontiers in Microbiology/Virology, 4*, 293. doi:10.3389/fmicb.2013.00293

Mangla, A. (2014). Brain-type natriuretic peptide (BNP). Retrieved from http://emedicine.medscape.com/article/2087425-overview

Maughan, B., Asselin, N., Carey, J., Sucov, A., & Valente, J. (2013). False-negative chest radiographs in emergency department diagnosis of pneumonia. *Rhode Island Medical Journal, 97*(8), 20–23.

Parikh, R., Seliger, S., & deFilippi, C. (2015). Use and interpretation of high sensitivity cardiac troponins in patients with chronic kidney disease with and without acute myocardial infarction. *Clinical Biochemistry, 48*(4–5), 247–253. doi:10.1016/j.clinbiochem.2015.01.004

Ponikowski, P., Voors, A., Anker, S., Bueno, H., Cleland, J., Coats, A., … van der Meer, P. (2016). 2016 ESC Guidelines for the diagnosis and treatment of acute and chronic heart failure: The Task Force for the diagnosis and treatment of acute and chronic heart failure of the European Society of Cardiology (ESC). *European Heart Journal, 37*(27), 2129–2200.

Romel, S., Faruque, M., Bari, M. A., Bari, M. S., Aditya, G., Choudhury, A., ... Alam, M. (2014). Association between elevated B-type natriuretic peptide levels with extent of coronary artery disease in patients with unstable angina and NSTEMI. *Mymensingh Medical Journal, 23*(3), 544–551.

Rosenberg, M. (2016, February 24). Overview of the management of chronic kidney disease in adults. Retrieved from http://www.uptodate.com/contents/overview-of-the-management-of-chronic-kidney-disease-in-adults?source+serarch_results&search=failure%20of%20disease%20adult&selectedtitle=2~150

Rui, P., Kang, K., & Albert, M. (2013). National Hospital Medical Care Survey: 2013 emergency department summary tables. Retrieved from http://www. cdc.gov/nchs/data/ahcd/nhamcs_emergency/2013_ed_web_tables. pdf

Segall, L., Nistor, I., & Covic, A. (2014). Heart failure in patients with chronic kidney disease: A systematic integrative review. *BioMed Research International, 2014*, article ID 937398. doi:10.1155/2014/937398

# CHAPTER 4

# Shortness of Breath: Another Encounter

The scenario that begins this chapter demonstrates variations in the history and the key features obtained by two different providers evaluating the same patient. As in Chapter 2, we focus on the initial interaction and interview between each provider and the patient. The pertinent pieces of history are then identified and compared.

## CASE SCENARIO

A 67-year-old White male who was recently diagnosed with stage 2 DLBCL was admitted to the hospital nearly 24 hours ago with neutropenic fever. He completed his first cycle of chemotherapy with R-CHOP (rituximab, cyclophosphamide, doxorubicin, vincristine, and prednisone) 12 days ago. He has been placed on appropriate antibiotic therapy and blood cultures are pending. An initial chest film showed bilateral pleural effusions, mild cardiomegaly, and hilar lymphadenopathy. He reported bilateral ankle swelling and was treated with 20 mg IV furosemide on admission. Around 11 a.m., however, he complains of shortness of breath. He is afebrile, but his heart rate has increased to 90 beats per minute from a baseline of 65 beats per minute, and his blood

*(continued)*

## CASE SCENARIO (*continued*)

pressure has slowly declined to 96/60 mmHg from 112/72 mmHg. The nurse notifies the HemOnc service about the change in the patient's condition.

DLBCL, diffuse large B-cell non-Hodgkin's lymphoma; HemOnc, hematology/oncology; IV, intravenous; R-CHOP, rituximab, cyclophosphamide, doxorubicin, vincristine, and prednisone.

The HemOnc fellow orders a stat chest film and comes to evaluate the patient. He asks the following questions:

Q: **How you are feeling right now?**

A: Not well. I'm having a hard time breathing.

Q: **When did this start?**

A: A little while ago—shortly after breakfast—around 9:30. I had a hard time walking around my room.

Q: **Does this feeling improve when you are sitting here in bed?**

A: A little, but I still feel like I can't get enough air.

Q: **Are you having any chest pain or dizziness?**

A: No chest pain. I was a little lightheaded when I was up moving about, but not now.

Q: **Any chills, nausea, or vomiting?**

A: No.

The chest film is completed. The HemOnc fellow reviews the image and notes no change from the prior film. An ECG is ordered that shows normal sinus rhythm with low voltage. The exam performed by the HemOnc fellow is notable for diminished lung and heart sounds, bilateral ankle edema, and elevated jugular venous pressure. Concerned that the patient is in heart failure, he orders oxygen; a stat complete blood count (CBC); chemistry panel; brain natriuretic peptide (BNP) and troponin levels; and an echocardiogram. Given the low blood pressure he is hesitant to order an additional dose of furosemide, so he calls the cardio-vascular clinician for consultation to assist in management of suspected acute heart failure.

The information presented to the consulting cardiovascular clinician is summarized in history A.

## HISTORY A

*A 67-year-old White male with a past medical history of hyperlipidemia and recently diagnosed with stage 2 DLBCL who completed his first cycle of RCHOP therapy 12 days ago was admitted yesterday with neutropenic fever, ankle edema, and bilateral pleural effusions. We initially treated him with furosemide and started empiric antibiotic therapy. Blood cultures are pending. He started to complain of shortness of breath this afternoon and has evidence of volume overload on exam. He denies any chest pain or associated symptoms, but feels lightheaded when ambulating. Labs are pending and chest film does not show improvement from yesterday. An ECG does not show any signs of ischemia based on my review. He has evidence of edema and jugular venous distention (JVD) on exam. His blood pressure has decreased making further diuresis more challenging. We are concerned he may have developed heart failure and possibly reduced ejection fraction due to the chemotherapy and we'd like cardiology assistance in managing this issue.*

The cardiovascular clinician immediately reviews the chart for other relevant data obtained since the patient was admitted yesterday. Is anything missing from the story that can help the consulting provider?

When asked to consult on any patient with a potential cardiac issue, it is important to identify any baseline data that may be available. In this case, the cardiovascular clinician should look for prior ECGs, echocardio-grams, chest films, and laboratory trends as well as current medications that may influence symptoms. This patient has been followed at this insti-tution for all of his care. No ECG was done on admission, but an ECG was done 2 months ago, along with an echocardiogram and a chest film. The results of these tests provide a great basis for comparison with current findings and are discussed later in the chapter.

The fluid balance should be noted whenever a patient is being treated for heart failure or has received a diuretic for any reason. This patient received furosemide, 20 mg intravenously, yesterday and had 1,200 mL of urine output, with his overall fluid balance being −1 L. The cardiovascular clinician wonders why the patient has not improved with this amount of diuresis.

As mentioned by the HemOnc fellow, the patient has received RCHOP therapy, which contains a well-known cardiotoxic agent, doxorubicin. The consultant next focuses on determining whether the patient is experiencing heart failure from possible chemotherapy-induced cardiomyopathy, or something more sinister.

Vital signs are obtained at the bedside, as follows: Blood pressure, 92/58 mmHg; pulse, 101 beats per minute; respiratory rate, 20 breaths per minute; and oxygen saturation, 95% on 2 L/minute of oxygen. The patient is afebrile. The cardiovascular clinician asks the patient the following questions:

Q: **How you are feeling right now?**

A: I'm really short of breath.

Q: **Describe it for me. Does it feel like you can't get a full breath or that you can't get enough air without breathing rapidly, or something else altogether?**

A: I feel like I can't get a good breath. It feels like a fullness in my chest—like I can't get enough air.

Q: **When did you first notice this?**

A: Earlier today, shortly after breakfast, around 9:30.

Q: **Did you have any shortness of breath when you first came to the hospital?**

A: Not really. I get tired and a little short of breath with too much activity, but I figure this is just from my cancer.

Q: **Do you feel like your symptoms are getting worse as the day goes on or are they staying about the same?**

A: I think they are getting worse. I'm short of breath sitting here.

Q: **Do you have any chest pain, pressure, or heaviness, or any back, jaw, or arm pain?**

A: No.

Q: **How has your urine output been? Do you feel like it has slowed down since yesterday?**

A: I went to the bathroom a lot after that dose of Lasix (furosemide), but I have hardly gone at all today.

Q: **Have you had swelling in your ankles, or increased abdominal fullness or bloating?**

A: My ankles have been swollen for the past 3 to 4 days.

Q: **Are they worse, better, or about the same now?**

A: About the same as when they first started swelling.

Q: **So you have not noticed any improvement since the Lasix was given?**

A: No, not really.

Q: **Are you lightheaded, dizzy, sweaty, nauseated, or having any cough?**

A: I was a lightheaded when I was up and about earlier in my room. Not now though. No cough.

Q: **Have you ever had a history of heart failure, heart attack, or blood clots to your lungs?**

A: No. I'm being treated for high cholesterol. Other than the lymphoma I've been healthy.

Q: **Have you noticed whether your shortness of breath gets worse if you lie flat?**

A: I do feel better sitting straight up like this.

Q: **Do you have any palpitations or the sensation that your heart is beating rapidly?**

A: No. I just don't feel well at all.

The cardiovascular clinician has thoroughly evaluated the patient's complaint of shortness of breath. The exam, which is also performed at this point, is detailed later in the chapter. The history of present illness is summarized in history B.

## HISTORY B

*A 67-year-old White male with a history of hyperlipidemia and a recent diagnosis of stage 2 DLBCL was admitted yesterday for neutropenic fever. He completed his first cycle of RCHOP 12 days ago. He had evidence of bilateral pleural effusions and ankle edema, which had been present for the past 4 days. He was started on empiric antibiotic therapy and given a dose of furosemide, 20 mg IV, upon arrival. Despite adequate urine output initially, he has had no improvement in symptoms and notices a decrease in urinary frequency presently.*

*Today he developed shortness of breath described as a feeling of fullness and inability to get air shortly after breakfast. He feels short of breath at rest and feels more comfortable in the upright position. He noted he was lightheaded with ambulation and has been mildly short of breath for the past few weeks with exertion only. He denies any chest pain, pressure, tightness, or any chest-related symptoms as well as any nausea, vomiting, diaphoresis, cough, or palpitations. His blood pressure has declined and he is now tachycardic. He has no history of heart attack, heart failure, or a blood clot to the lungs.*

*Initial evaluation by the primary service was concerning for acute heart failure. A chest film was unchanged from admission and notable for cardiomegaly. There is concern that he may have developed a chemotherapy-induced cardiomyopathy and, due to his low blood pressure with the possible need for further diuresis, cardiology has been asked to assist in management.*

Now remember, although an exam has been completed at this point by the cardiovascular clinician, and other data have been reviewed, this is merely a summary of the patient's chief complaint. Without any additional information, does this seem like a picture of heart failure?

You should be considering all the other acute conditions in addition to heart failure at this point based on the background information and symptoms.

## KEY FEATURES OF THE HISTORY

The history obtained by each provider is somewhat different in this case. The patient had already been admitted and what was his initial complaint is not the primary issue at present. When there is an acute change in the patient's condition relevant information needs to be gathered quickly to determine the next best course of action. Let us review the key features of history A and history B and compare how each provider obtained them in order to determine whether the primary diagnosis is the same.

## Character

Character was identified in history A and history B by asking the patient what he was feeling. He expressed that he was having a hard time breathing. The consulting cardiovascular clinician went on to ask more specific questions about the nature of his shortness of breath, that is, whether it felt as if he could not get a full breath or was unable to get enough air. The patient responded that it felt like fullness in his chest and that he could not get enough air. Differentiating between the characteristics of shortness of breath is challenging, but the perception of fullness is an important detail.

The cardiovascular clinician also asked the patient whether his symptoms were present on admission and if they were getting worse or staying the same. He responded that he felt they were getting worse and that he was short of breath just sitting in the bed. He did note that he had been short of breath with activity before admission but did not feel this was relevant to the current symptoms. He felt it was related to his primary diagnosis.

Establishing the presence of symptoms previously is important when trying to consider differential diagnoses in which shortness of breath can be progressive or acute. In history A, the first provider also asked if the patient's symptoms were improved with rest but did not ask whether he had them at all at the time of admission.

## Timing and Duration

Both clinicians asked when the symptoms started, and the patient's response was the same. Both were able to identify that the symptoms were first noted on ambulation in the room and are now present at rest as well. Initially the patient told the HemOnc fellow he felt a little improvement with rest, but he later told the cardiology provider he felt as though he was getting worse—even at rest.

Time had elapsed between each evaluation, which can certainly alter the patient's responses; the subtle notation of progression speaks not only to the severity of symptoms but also to the duration. This patient has had no relief of symptoms, which are ongoing—this is evident from both histories. One other factor that should be considered in relation to timing is when the patient's chemotherapy was completed and whether it is related to his symptoms. Cardiotoxicity can be acute and can occur even within 24 hours of dosing (Octavia et al., 2012). This patient completed his first cycle of RCHOP therapy 12 days ago, so the connection between this regimen and his symptoms must be considered when seeking to determine a cause.

## Associated Symptoms

The HemOnc fellow asked the patient whether he was having chest pain or dizziness, chills, nausea, or vomiting. The consulting cardiovascular clinician also asked these questions but expanded the questioning of chest pain to ask about chest tightness or heaviness, and jaw, back, or arm pain. Both providers were able to elicit that the patient was lightheaded upon ambulating but not in the bed.

The patient presented on admission with swollen ankles, which were documented but not queried directly by the first provider. The second provider asked about swelling, abdominal fullness, or bloating. The first provider relayed the fact that the patient had edema on exam, and the patient confirmed with the second provider that his ankles remained swollen without improvement. The second provider also asked whether the patient was experiencing palpitations. Palpitations can contribute to the perception of shortness of breath, so this was an important associated symptom about which to inquire. However, both providers were able to determine that the only associated symptom was lightheadedness with ambulation.

## Mitigating or Alleviating Factors

The first provider did not ask the patient directly if anything made his shortness of breath better or worse. The statement made by the patient that he felt some improvement sitting in the bed was the only alleviating factor obtained.

The second provider asked the patient whether lying flat worsened his symptoms, and the patient responded that he was more comfortable sitting forward. The relationship of position to shortness of breath is important. The differential diagnoses of shortness of breath are vast, as we have documented, but only a few are associated with orthopnea, so this is a key piece of information. The second provider also asked more questions about the furosemide that was given on admission and how it related to the patient's ankle edema and symptoms, as well as asking about urine output. If a diuretic is given to a patient and he or she has adequate or copious amounts of output, the symptoms should improve. The fact that the diuretic did not alleviate his symptoms and, in fact, may have worsened them should lead your thinking to a diagnosis other than heart failure.

# KEY FEATURES OF THE DATA

The key features of the data relevant to this scenario are the vital signs; past and present imaging, which includes echocardiogram, chest films, and ECGs; and, less importantly, laboratory findings.

## Vital Signs

The following findings are reported at the time the cardiovascular clinician evaluates the patient:

*Blood pressure:* Initially 92/58 mmHg; it is retaken on both arms—
   Right arm 90/54 mmHg, left arm 88/56 mmHg

*Pulse:* 101 to 109 beats per minute

*Respirations:* 20 breaths per minute

*Oxygen saturation:* 95% on 2 L/min of oxygen

*Temperature:* 36.5°C

Since this patient was admitted the previous day, trends in vital signs are reviewed. On admission, the patient's blood pressures ranged from 112/72 to 126/68 mmHg. His pulse around the time of admission was around 65 beats per minute. His respiratory rate was 14 breaths per minute and his temperature was 38.4°C on admission, 38.0°C on the next reading, but normal thereafter. He is clearly tachypneic, tachycardic, and hypotensive. Intake and output balance since admission is reviewed. He had 1,200 mL of urine output and has an overall fluid balance of –1 L. Fluid balance is critical when assessing response to diuretic therapy.

## Electrocardiogram (ECG)

The patient did not have an ECG upon admission. One was obtained urgently when the patient was initially evaluated by the HemOnc fellow and was reported to be normal without evidence of ischemic findings. The patient did have an ECG 2 months ago. It was read as normal sinus rhythm with a heart rate of 68 beats per minute. No ST segment or T-wave abnormalities were noted.

The ECG done today shows a reduction in voltage and evidence of electrical alternans. Heart rate is 95 beats per minute and there are no ST segment or T-wave abnormalities. On initial review, the low voltage and electrical alternans may not have been noticeable to the HemOnc fellow, particularly if the ECG was not compared to a prior one. For a cardiovascular clinician, however, it is imperative to review the ECGs for any cardiac abnormalities that may present with electrocardiographic findings. Pericardial effusion or pericardial tamponade should be considered whenever electrical alternans are seen on an ECG (Jehangir & Osman, 2015).

## Echocardiogram

This patient underwent echocardiography 2 months ago before beginning chemotherapy. According to current guidelines it is standard to have a baseline assessment of cardiac function prior to initiating chemotherapy, particularly when potentially cardiotoxic agents will be used (Plana et al., 2014). This patient is undergoing RCHOP therapy, which contains doxorubicin—an agent well known to have potential adverse effects on cardiac function.

The echocardiogram obtained 2 months ago showed normal left ventricular size and function with an ejection fraction of 66%. Right ventricular size and function were normal, and there were no atrial or valvular abnormalities. The patient was noted to have a tiny pericardial effusion. A repeat echocardiogram has been ordered but has not yet been obtained.

Do you have a suspicion of what it might show? During the evaluation, the cardiovascular clinician should consider the possibility of a reduced ejection fraction and perhaps a pericardial effusion. The results of this study can be crucial in the treatment of this patient's symptoms.

## Chest Radiograph

The chest film from 2 months ago was reviewed. On that study, the cardiac silhouette was normal. There were small pleural effusions as well as bilateral hilar lymphadenopathy. No other pulmonary process or edema was noted. The chest film on admission did reveal bilateral pleural effusions, some mild cardiomegaly, and again the hilar lymphadenopathy consistent with his lymphoma.

A repeat chest film was obtained urgently at the time the patient reported a change in symptoms. The first provider reported no change from the film on admission, but only the findings specific to the lungs might have been reviewed. The cardiovascular clinician did a side-by-side comparison of the two studies and noted that cardiomegaly was somewhat more pronounced and the heart appeared globular. The pleural effusions were unchanged. The formal report noted the worsening appearance of cardiomegaly.

## Biomarkers and Lab Results

The troponin T level was less than 0.01 ng/mL. The patient's symptoms began around 9:30 a.m., and the troponin level was drawn just before 12 p.m. As we have learned in earlier chapters, the troponin level does not rise for at least 3 to 4 hours after myocardial injury (Mangla & Gupta, 2015). A negative value is reassuring, but it does not yet exclude ischemia.

The CBC was reviewed and the white blood cell (WBC) count was noted to still be low at 1,078. This is improved from the admission value of 890. Hemoglobin at the time of patient's diagnosis 2 months ago was 11.4 g/dL. On admission, this value was 9.6 g/dL, and it is currently stable at 9.4 g/dL. Platelet count was within the low normal range 2 months ago, but on admission platelets were 70,000 and they are currently 76,000. It is well documented that anemia can cause shortness of breath; however, it is unlikely the primary cause of this patient's symptoms considering that his hemoglobin has been relatively stable since admission.

A BNP level was drawn and noted to be 98 pg/mL. A D-dimer level was not drawn with the rationale that it might lead to a false positive result given the lack of specificity in the setting of malignancy in this case (Kabrhel et al., 2013). The chemistry panel was notable for a creatinine level of 1.4 mg/dL. On admission, the creatinine was 1.1 mg/dL and the patient's baseline from prior review was between 0.8 mg/dL and 1.0 mg/dL.

Could an acute kidney injury be causing the patient's symptoms, or are they occurring in response to such injury? Diuretics can be associated with an acute kidney injury (Ejaz & Mohandas, 2014). If diuretics are used there is the expectation that overall volume loss will occur with reduction in effusions, edema, and improved symptoms. When excessive diuresis occurs, urine output can decrease and kidney function can decline (Singh & Sabath, 2016). This patient had no improvement of symptoms despite adequate urine output that did not exceed expectations with the use of furosemide. So why does this patient seem to be having increasing shortness of breath?

## Other Data

The patient's current medications are reviewed. He is on atorvastatin, 40 mg at night; heparin, subcutaneously, 5,000 units every 12 hours; omeprazole, 20 mg daily; and piperacillin/tazobactam, 4.5g intravenously every 6 hours. His only other medical history outside of his recent diagnosis of non-Hodgkin's lymphoma is hyperlipidemia.

The cardiovascular clinician asked about any history of heart attacks, blood clots, or heart failure, which he denied. He is a lifelong nonsmoker. He does not drink or use illicit drugs. He was very active before his diagnosis of lymphoma. His family history is unremarkable for premature coronary artery disease, cardiomyopathies, or cancers. He is at low risk for coronary artery disease, but it must still be considered as an underlying mechanism for his symptoms, although perhaps less likely.

# DIFFERENTIALS AND DIFFERENCES IN EXAM

The exam in this patient should focus on looking for anything that might support the working diagnosis or discount it. Once again, the chest, lungs, abdomen, and extremities should be thoroughly evaluated. The focus should be on evidence of volume overload, any adventitious findings on auscultation, and signs of perfusion or lack thereof.

The cardiovascular clinician performs an exam and the findings are as follows:

*General appearance:* Thin-appearing White male in a moderate amount of distress.

*Head and neck:* Head is normocephalic and atraumatic, without evidence of lesions or masses. Sclera are anicteric. Neck is soft and supple, without thyromegaly. Supraclavicular and cervical lymphadenopathy are present.

*Cardiac exam:* Jugular venous pressure is elevated to the level of the earlobe. No carotid bruits. No abdominal or femoral bruits. Peripheral pulses are palpable and symmetric. Loss of peripheral pulse is noted on inspiration. Auscultation of the heart reveals distant heart sounds, S1 and S2 present. No S3 or S4. No murmurs, heaves, rubs, or lifts. Chest wall is nontender to palpation.

*Lungs:* Reduced sounds in bases bilaterally with faint crackles. Symmetric expansion.

*Abdomen:* Soft, nontender. Bowel sounds present in all four quadrants.

*Extremities:* Skin cool but dry. There is 2+ pitting edema noted bilaterally in the pretibial and ankle regions. No clubbing or cyanosis.

*Neurological:* Alert and oriented ×3. Cranial nerves are intact. Motor strength is symmetric in bilateral upper and lower extremities. Sensation is intact. No focal neurological deficits.

The exam performed by both providers revealed evidence of edema and JVD. One other important clinical exam finding was uncovered by the cardiovascular clinician: the loss of pulse with inspiration. This is a quick bedside assessment that is equivalent to pulsus paradoxus.

When this was noted, the consulting provider obtained another blood pressure reading and determined that this patient had pulsus paradoxus of 36 mmHg.

Now that we can combine the history with other key data and the physical exam, do you still think this patient is in acute heart failure?

This patient had the presence of Beck's triad, which is:

- Hypotension
- Muffled heart sounds
- Elevated jugular venous pressure

All of these findings are present in cardiac tamponade (LeWinter & Hopkins, 2015). These physical findings along with electrical alternans with low voltage on ECG and the chest film should make you think of cardiac tamponade as the primary diagnosis, not heart failure. This diagnosis is one that must be identified and treated urgently as it can be life threatening.

Enough information is available in this case that is consistent with a presentation of cardiac tamponade to indicate that treatment of that condition should be pursued without further consideration of other possible causes for shortness of breath.

Let us review the differential diagnosis list we developed in Chapter 3, examining these conditions in relation to the patient's chief complaint to explore how the final diagnosis was made.

### Differential Diagnoses of Shortness of Breath

| | | |
|---|---|---|
| • Anaphylaxis | • interstitial lung disease | • Pneumonia/respiratory infection |
| • Cardiac tamponade | • Lung cancer | • Pulmonary embolus |
| • COPD/asthma exacerbation | • Myocardial infarction | • Pneumothorax |
| • Heart failure | • (PAH) | • Unstable angina |

COPD, Chronic obstructive pulmonary disease; PAH, Pulmonary arterial hypertension.

# PULLING IT ALL TOGETHER

## Working Through the Differential

We can eliminate a few diagnoses right away. Anaphylaxis, pneumothorax, and COPD/asthma exacerbation can all be taken off our differential diagnosis list. The history of present illness and objective data do not support these diagnoses.

PAH was not present on the echocardiogram performed 2 months ago. It can sometimes be hard to differentiate features of PAH from those of heart failure with preserved ejection fraction of 50% or greater (HFpEF; McLaughlin & Humbert, 2015). While this may be a possibility, it is unlikely the primary underlying diagnosis causing his symptoms. Patients with PAH who have cardiac tamponade typically do not have the common features of pulsus paradoxus and hypotension (Sahay & Tonelli, 2013). The echocardiogram will certainly confirm this as unlikely, but it is safe to move it lower on our differential list.

Pneumonia or other respiratory infection is less likely given the other associated features, such as the nature of his shortness of breath and the absence of overt infection on the chest film. He is already receiving antibiotic therapy for the neutropenic fever and, while this is a concern, it is not the cause of his current presentation.

This patient is at high risk for pulmonary embolus because of his history of cancer. Cancer patients have a four- to sevenfold increased risk of symptomatic venous thromboembolism and a five- to sevenfold increased risk of bleeding on anticoagulation (Liebman & O'Connell, 2016). The patient has dyspnea and tachycardia, but no chest pain, and he has been receiving heparin prophylaxis during his hospitalization. As discussed previously, a D-dimer test may not be helpful in this situation, but the patient will likely not be able to lie flat for a CT scan. This creates a diagnostic dilemma.

While pulmonary embolus is certainly a possibility, the positive pulsus finding, JVD, and globular appearance of the heart on chest film are most consistent with cardiac tamponade, and confirming this diagnosis is more important than ruling out a pulmonary embolus. The treatment for pulmonary embolus is anticoagulation; however, treating this patient empirically with anticoagulation without proof could cause hemopericardium and worsening of the suspected effusion.

Interstitial lung disease is also less likely given the presence of edema and hemodynamic changes that have occurred more acutely. The chest film was not suspicious for this. Certainly, a CT scan of the chest would aid further evaluation; however, it is safe to eliminate this diagnosis from our top differential list. Lung cancer is a possibility but would not cause the objective findings noted in this patient.

What about myocardial infarction or unstable angina? Before his diagnosis of lymphoma, this patient was very active and his only risk factor for coronary artery disease is hyperlipidemia. His baseline echocardiogram did not reveal any wall motion abnormalities suggestive of myocardial ischemia at that time. The ECG obtained when his symptoms began did not show evidence of ischemia, and the troponin level is undetectable.

Some studies have reported an increased risk of heart failure, cardiomyopathy, and acute myocardial infarctions in DLBCL patients receiving doxorubicin-based therapy who did not have a prior history of cardiovascular disease (Tsai, Pfeiffer, Warren, Wilson, & Landgren, 2015). It is possible an acute ischemic event could be causing shortness of breath and edema, but it is certainly not our number one differential given the exam findings and lack of ischemic findings on ECG.

The two diagnoses left on the list are heart failure and cardiac tamponade. Shortness of breath, edema, JVD, and hypotension can all be symptoms of both. As we have noted, doxorubicin therapy can cause cardiomyopathy. The timing can vary from acutely to many years later, so it remains a lifelong concern (Octavia et al., 2012). It was also reasonable in this case to presume that heart failure from new-onset cardiomyopathy was causing this patient's symptoms, given the cardiomegaly on chest film.

The interesting point to highlight in this scenario is that the patient's symptoms worsened with diuresis rather than improving, as one would expect when treating edema from heart failure. Why would this be?

First, slow accumulation of pericardial fluid over time can be well tolerated and can result in edema. Rapid accumulation of fluid can lead to sudden hypotension and cause cardiac tamponade even with lower amounts of fluid in the pericardial space. This patient had a small effusion on his echocardiogram 2 months ago, so it is reasonable to assume this effusion was slowly accumulating. He also reported shortness of breath with activity leading up to his admission. This is consistent with a slower accumulation of fluid.

Second, diuretics can worsen cardiac tamponade by removing enough volume from the circulation to lower central venous pressure below intrapericardial pressure (Schiavone, 2013). This would explain why this patient, who had likely been compensating for some time, decompensated with diuresis. The rise in his creatinine level might also have contributed to overdiuresis initially, but that combined with the reduction in urine output and hypotension was likely a consequence of the pericardial effusion rather than a prerenal acute kidney injury (Sing & Sabath, 2016).

This patient's treatment with a potentially cardiotoxic chemotherapeutic drug put him at risk for heart failure, but his neoplastic process also puts him at risk for pericardial effusion and potential cardiac tamponade. Lymphomas can occasionally cause effusion in association with enlarged mediastinal lymph nodes by obstructing lymph drainage (LeWinter & Hopkins, 2015).

Although his symptoms are similar to those noted in heart failure, another differentiation is the presence of electrical alternans and low voltage on ECG as well as pulsus paradoxus—key features in cardiac tamponade. Shortness of breath is the most common complaint in patients with cardiac tamponade, having a sensitivity of 87% to 88% (Fang & O'Gara, 2015). Further, hypotension and muffled heart sounds can also be present—and this patient had both. Confirming this diagnosis with echocardiography is imperative so the patient can be treated urgently before further hemodynamic compromise or cardiac arrest ensues.

**Likely Diagnosis:** Cardiac tamponade

---

## WHAT'S NEXT?

- Once cardiac tamponade is suspected, a liter of normal saline is infused rapidly to maintain intravascular volume and avoid ventricular collapse.

- An urgent echocardiogram confirms a moderate to large circumferential pericardial effusion with tamponade physiology and a preserved ejection fraction of 68%.

- The patient is taken urgently to the cardiac catheterization lab for ultrasound-guided pericardiocentesis and drain placement.

- Approximately 800 mL of straw-colored fluid is drained. Cytologic evaluation of the fluid to determine whether it is malignant or infectious comes back negative.

- Blood pressure, creatinine levels, and urine output immediately return to normal following the procedure.

## SUMMARIZING THE SCENARIO

This clinical case was challenging because the history obtained from the patient could not clearly identify the primary diagnosis. History and physical exam findings perform poorly as independent predictors of pericardial effusions (Stolz et al., 2017). Once the effusion is significant enough to cause cardiac tamponade, however, the physical exam findings can be critical in differentiating this from other diagnoses.

Pericardial effusions and subsequent cardiac tamponade do not occur spontaneously in normally healthy individuals. This patient's background of DLBCL with mediastinal involvement, recent chemotherapy, and prior (albeit small) effusion were helpful in identifying his risk of developing tamponade in this setting. His history also placed him at higher risk of developing heart failure, which prompted the initial consideration. If the ECG had been more carefully examined, or evaluation for pulsus paradoxus had been done by the first provider—the diagnosis of cardiac tamponade might have been identified sooner allowing for even more rapid treatment.

When evaluating a specific subset of patients such as this one, we must consider what risk factors are involved for developing a life-threatening condition that we may not typically encounter in our patients. In this case, there were few differentiating features in the histories obtained by each provider, and ultimately it was the physical exam findings that led to the diagnosis.

The positional component of the patient's shortness of breath along with the feeling of "fullness" and the lack of improvement with diuresis were important factors identified by the second provider that directed the clinical suspicion to something other than heart failure. Rapid infusion of intravascular volume in any patient with suspected cardiac tamponade can be lifesaving until drainage can be achieved. The prompt recognition by the cardiovascular clinician and initiation of IV fluids likely avoided further hemodynamic compromise in this patient.

## COMMON PITFALLS AND ASSUMPTIONS

Shortness of breath can indicate a wide variety of diseases and can often be a consequence of a primary process that may not seem related initially. It can be challenging as a provider to determine whether a patient's symptoms represent tightness, air hunger, suffocation, breathlessness, or something else. These are subtle details that can help narrow the differential.

Patients with this complaint are often in distress, and obtaining key details can be difficult. That is why it is important that any other relevant data related to timing, associated factors, and background information be gathered to ensure an accurate picture. Any positional component or factors such as orthopnea, edema, palpitations, and syncope or chest pain can help to delineate a primary cause.

The nature of this complaint calls for prompt treatment to alleviate symptoms—sometimes before all the necessary information can be gathered. Evaluation of a patient with shortness of breath is an ongoing process, and treatment should be modified as data are gathered to correct the underlying cause as well as improve symptoms. It is important to differentiate the two. Treatment of shortness of breath often involves oxygen supplementation or positive pressure ventilation to avoid respiratory failure, but this does not necessarily mean the root cause is identified by these actions. They may lead to improvement of symptoms, but further investigation needs to continue to restore the patient to baseline function, if possible.

The case scenarios presented in this chapter and in Chapter 3 demonstrate a complaint of shortness of breath that was treated based on an incorrect or presumed diagnosis. The detailed history obtained by the cardiovascular clinician in the scenario in Chapter 3 led to an alternative diagnosis of non-ST-elevation myocardial infarction (NSTEMI) rather than heart failure and cardiac tamponade, as was the case in the current scenario.

All patients with shortness of breath and edema do not necessarily have heart failure, and typical treatment with diuretics is not always indicated. Such treatment can, in some cases, worsen the condition, as demonstrated in the current case. In addition, an elevated BNP does not always correlate with heart failure, and other causes must be considered in relation to the clinical picture.

We also learned in Chapter 3 that patients with coronary ischemia do not always present with chest pain, particularly in the case of women and diabetics, so the absence of this symptom does not necessarily rule out this diagnosis. The presence of risk factors for certain diagnoses, other comorbid conditions, and treatment of those conditions all must be considered when determining the potential causes of a patient's symptoms.

The history obtained by the cardiovascular clinician in the current scenario was slightly more detailed than that of the first provider, but it did not dismiss a diagnosis of heart failure. An assumption was made by the first provider based on the classic signs of heart failure, and an alternative diagnosis was not immediately considered. We cannot make any assumptions though, because things are not always what they appear to be. In this case it was the astute clinical exam with the consideration of underlying malignancy and risk for cardiac tamponade that led to the right diagnosis.

To summarize, any patient presenting with a chief complaint of shortness of breath must be evaluated, examined, and treated quickly to avoid further distress or cardiorespiratory arrest. The setting in which the symptom has occurred, the timing, and any associated factors are the most important features when seeing a patient with this complaint. Any acute differential diagnosis must be identified or eliminated quickly. To do so, the clinician must ask the necessary questions and perform the exam with this approach in mind.

# REFERENCES

Ejaz, A., & Mohandas, R. (2014). Are diuretics harmful in the management of acute kidney injury? *Current Opinion in Nephrology and Hypertension*, *23*(2), 155–160.

Fang, J., & O-Gara, P. (2015). The history and physical examination: An evidence-based approach. In *Braunwald's heart disease: A textbook of cardiovascular medicine* (10th ed.). Philadelphia, PA: Elsevier/Saunders.

Jehangir, W., & Osman, M. (2015). Electrical alternans with pericardial tamponade. *New England Journal of Medicine, 373*, e10.

Kabrhel, C., Courtney, D., Camargo Jr., C., Plewa, M., Nordenholz, K., Moore, C., ... Kline, J. (2010). Factors associated with positive D-dimer results in patients evaluated for pulmonary embolism. *Academic Emergency Medicine, 17*(6), 589–597. doi:10.1111/j.1553-2712.2010.00765.x

LeWinter, M., & Hopkins, W. (2015). Pericardial diseases. In *Braunwald's heart disease: A textbook of cardiovascular medicine* (10th ed.). Philadelphia, PA: Elsevier/Saunders.

Liebman, H., & O'Connell, C. (2016). Incidental venous thromboembolic events in cancer patients: What we know in 2016. *Thrombosis Research, 140*(1), s18–s20.

Mangla, A., & Gupta, A. (2015). Troponins. Retrieved from http://emedicine.medscape.com/article/2073935-overview

McLaughlin, V., & Humbert, M. (2015). Pulmonary hypertension. In D. L. Mann, D. P. Zipes, P. Libby, & R. O. Bonow, *Braunwald's heart disease: A textbook of cardiovascular medicine* (10th ed., pp. 1682–1702). Philadelphia, PA: Elsevier/Saunders.

Octavia, Y., Tocchetti, C., Gabrielson, K., Janssens, S., Crijns, H., & Moens, A. (2012). Doxorubicin-induced cardiomyopathy: From molecular mechanisms to therapeutic strategies. *Journal of Molecular and Cellular Cardiology, 52*, 1213–1225.

Plana, J., Galderisi, M., Barac, A., Ewer, M., Ky, B., Scherrer-Crosbie, M., ... Lancellotti, P. (2014). Expert consensus for multimodality imaging evaluation of adult patients during and after cancer therapy: A report from the American Society of Echocardiography and the European Association of Cardiovascular Imaging. *Journal of the American Society of Echocardiography, 27*, 911–939.

Sahay, S., & Tonelli, A. (2013). Pericardial effusion in pulmonary arterial hypertension. *Pulmonary Circulation, 3*(3), 467–477. doi:10.1086/674302

Schiavone, W. (2013). Cardiac tamponade: 12 pearls in diagnosis and management. *Cleveland Clinic Journal of Medicine, 80*(2), 109–116.

Singh, G., & Sabath, B., (2016). Over-diuresis or cardiac tamponade? An unusual case of acute kidney injury and early closure. *Journal of Community Hospital Internal Medicine Perspectives, 6*, 31357. doi:10.3402/jchimp.v6.31357

Stolz, L., Valenzuela, J., Situ-LaCasse, E., Stolz, U., Hawbaker, N., Thompson, M., & Adhikari, S. (2017). Clinical and historical features of emergency department patients with pericardial effusions. *World Journal of Emergency Medicine*, *8*(1), 29–33, doi:10.5848/wjem.j.1920-8642.2017.01.005

Tsai, H., Pfeiffer, R., Warren, J., Wilson, W., & Landgren, O. (2015). The effects of cardiovascular disease on the clinical outcome of elderly patients with diffuse large B-cell lymphoma. *Leukemia & Lymphoma*, *56*(3), 682–687. doi:10.3109/10428194.2014.921914

# CHAPTER 5

# Syncope: A First Look

## DEFINITION AND SIGNIFICANCE OF SYNCOPE

According to the Farlex Partner Medical Dictionary (2012), syncope is defined as a "loss of consciousness and postural tone caused by diminished cerebral blood flow." This is not to be confused with what some patients refer to as "near fainting" or "lightheadedness," neither of which involves an actual loss of consciousness. Some sources further define syncope as a "transient loss of consciousness with return to baseline neurological function without medical intervention" (Patel & Quinn, 2015).

Syncope is a symptom and not a diagnosis. The causes can range from relatively benign to life threatening. Evaluating a patient with syncope can be challenging because there may not be a witness to describe what took place during the period of unconsciousness. In addition, patients often do not remember events or feelings leading up to the episode. A thorough history and specific exam findings can help in determining whether the syncopal spell was caused by a life-threatening diagnosis.

It is estimated that 1% to 2% of all emergency department visits result from a chief complaint of syncope; this is equivalent to approximately 1 million patients per year (Patel & Quinn, 2015). Approximately half of these patients are admitted to the hospital for further testing; the other half are discharged home without a clear diagnosis.

Many patients experience multiple syncopal events and, lacking a clear diagnosis, suffer negative impacts on their quality of life and mental health. Often patients who have had a syncopal episode are restricted from driving for a period of time, particularly if no diagnosis is made (Guzman & Morillo, 2015). This restriction, and ongoing uncertainty, can lead to feelings of depression, frustration, and discouragement.

Syncope is a symptom that often gets the attention of specialists in both neurology and cardiology. This is because many of the more serious diagnoses that can cause syncope are due to a neurological or cardiovascular condition. There are three major classifications of syncope (Saklani, Krahn, & Klein, 2013):

1. Reflex (neurally mediated) syncope—the most common type (vasovagal, situational, carotid sinus syncope)

2. Cardiac—the second most common types (arrhythmias, structural abnormalities)

3. Orthostatic syncope (volume depletion, autonomic dysfunction, drug induced)

Let us look at the following case scenario and once again examine how differences in the history can lead to different diagnoses.

## CASE SCENARIO

It is 5 p.m. and the cardiovascular clinician has been asked to consult on a patient who presented to the emergency department after an episode of syncope. The emergency physician is concerned that the patient's syncope may be caused by symptomatic bradycardia. History A is the initial history obtained by the emergency physician. History B is taken by the cardiovascular clinician. The emergency physician summarizes the information and communicates it to the consulting clinician and also states that the physical exam was unremarkable for any pertinent findings.

## HISTORY A

*A 47-year-old White female presented to the emergency department around 1600 after experiencing an episode of syncope. She has no significant past medical history and recently started running to train for her first half marathon. The episode today occurred around 2 p.m. today—about 30 minutes after she completed a 3-mile run. She was inside her home and reported feeling lightheaded. She attempted to sit down and as she was doing so, she passed out. Her husband was there and was able to ease her to the floor so she sustained no injuries. He reported there were no jerking movements or what he would perceive as "seizure-like" activity. He called her name and attempted to wake her. He did not feel for a pulse. He believes she was unconscious for about 1 minute. The patient does not recall the episode, but notes she felt "okay" when she came to. She denies any loss of bladder or bowel function. She has never experienced a syncopal event before today. She thought she might have been dehydrated, but her husband was concerned and insisted on bringing her in for further evaluation.*

Available data thus far are as follows:

## VITAL SIGNS

*Blood pressure*: 123/54 mmHg

*Pulse*: 45 beats per minute

*Respirations*: 14 breaths per minute

*Oxygen saturation*: 98% on room air

*Temperature*: 37.0°C

### Biomarkers, Lab Results, and Diagnostic Tests

The patient's CBC and chemistry panel show no abnormalities. The troponin T level is undetectable, and her chest film does not show any acute process. Her D-dimer level is within normal range. Her ECG is notable for bradycardia and a pattern of bigeminy with heart rate as previously noted. She is on no medications but takes calcium supplements, and vitamins $B_{12}$ and D.

---

CBC, complete blood count.

Based on the information available to you, what do you think is causing her syncope? Do you agree that she is having symptomatic bradycardia?

The cardiovascular clinician quickly assimilates the information provided and begins to examine the patient to gain further insight into the syncopal event and determine if bradycardia is in fact the cause. Symptomatic bradycardia is unusual in a woman of this age, so the clinician is already thinking of other possible differentials. After thoroughly evaluating the patient, the cardiovascular clinician summarizes the patient's presentation in history B.

## HISTORY B

*A 47-year-old White female with no significant past medical history presented to the emergency department this afternoon after experiencing an episode of syncope. The patient is physically active and recently began training for her first half marathon. She ran 3 miles today and about 30 minutes later experienced lightheadedness, palpitations, and the feeling she was going to "pass out." This was around 2 p.m. She attempted to sit down in a chair and, according to her husband, became limp and lost consciousness. He was able to catch her and ease her down to the floor. She sustained no injuries. Her husband states there was no seizure-like activity or jerking movements. He did not check for a pulse but called her name and touched her face in an attempt to wake her, without success. Her husband states it happened very quickly but believes she was only "out" for about a minute.*

*When the patient awoke she was aware of her surroundings, able to move all extremities, and had no memory of the actual event. She denies any loss of bowel or bladder control. She has never had a syncopal episode prior to today, but does report she has felt palpitations and lightheadedness on prior occasions, usually during and after she exercises. She felt all of these episodes were related to dehydration and has made it a point to drink a lot of water with these activities.*

*She denies experiencing any chest pain, arm pain, jaw pain, or back pain today or prior to today. She denies any fatigue, nausea, or vomiting. She reports shortness of breath and mild chest tightness with extreme exertion that starts halfway through her exercise and remains for a short period after, but has assumed it to be related to the fact she has just started running and feels she is simply "out of shape."*

*She notes her heart rate gets as high as 180 to 190 beats per minute when she feels these symptoms and takes a while to get back down to her baseline of 50 to 60 beats per minute even after she stops. She first noticed these symptoms about 1 month ago when she started running. She had these symptoms today toward the end of her run when she was sprinting. She denies symptoms consistent with orthostasis. She denies any orthopnea, paroxysmal nocturnal dyspnea, edema, or weight gain. She had a total hysterectomy 6 months ago for uterine fibroids and ovarian cysts and has intentionally lost weight since that time through dieting and exercise.*

*She has noted that lately she gets fatigued if she eats a large meal and experiences palpitations with this, as well. She was adopted as a child and has no information about her family history. Currently she feels that everything is back to her baseline and voices no complaints or concerns.*

Based on this history, do you think this patient was having symptomatic bradycardia or something else?

# KEY FEATURES OF THE HISTORY

History A and history B include all of the information gathered at the time each provider evaluated the patient. Both providers were thorough and identified pertinent information related to the patient's presenting symptom. The history taken by the cardiovascular clinician was more detailed and encompassed symptoms that the patient had at various times leading up to this event, which are relevant and will help to determine the right diagnosis.

Let us break down the information once again and compare the key features of the chief complaint of syncope.

## Character

The provider in history A identified the character of the chief complaint of syncope by asking the following questions:

Q: **What happened today that prompted you to come into the emergency department?**

A: I passed out.

Q: **What were you doing when this happened?**

A: I had just finished running 3 miles.

Q: **Did you feel it coming on—meaning, did you feel dizzy or lightheaded before?**

A: Yes, I felt lightheaded. I tried to sit down and then next thing I knew, I woke up on the floor.

Q: **Did you hurt yourself or was anyone around to see this?**

A: I did not hurt myself. My husband was there and apparently he caught me before I fell.

Q: **[To husband] Did you witness any jerking movements or seizure-like activity when she was unconscious?**

A: [Husband] No.

Q: **[To husband] Did you check for breathing or a pulse?**

A: [Husband] It happened very quickly, and she was awake before I thought about that. I just kept saying her name to try and get her to come around.

Q: **When you woke up, how did you feel? Had you lost bladder or bowel control?**

A: I felt okay. I didn't remember passing out. I did not lose bladder or bowel control.

Q: **Have you ever passed out before?**

A: No.

The cardiovascular clinician asked the following questions regarding the character of her syncope:

Q: **Why did you come to the emergency department today?**

A: I passed out.

Q: **What were you doing when this occurred?**

A: I had just finished a 3-mile run.

Q: Did you have any symptoms of dizziness, lightheadedness, palpitations, or chest pain or tightness before this event?

A: I felt lightheaded and I did have palpitations, maybe some mild tightness in my chest, as well. I was attempting to sit down and the next thing I knew I was on the floor with my husband next to me.

Q: [To husband] Did you witness this event? What did you see?

A: [Husband] I could tell she wasn't feeling well. I went over to her as she was trying to sit down and she went limp. I caught her and helped her to the floor and started calling her name and rubbing her face.

Q: [To husband] Did you notice any jerking or seizure-like activity?

A: [Husband] No.

Q: [To husband] Were you able to check a pulse?

A: [Husband] No. It happened very fast and I didn't even think to do that.

Q: [To husband] How long was she unconscious?

A: [Husband] I think it was about a minute, maybe less.

Q: Did you hit your head or sustain any injuries in your fall?

A: No.

Q: How did you feel when you woke up? Any confusion or loss of bowel or bladder control?

A: I felt okay. I did not remember passing out, but I did not lose bladder or bowel control.

Q: Have you ever had an episode like this before where you passed out or had the sensation that you were going to pass out?

A: I have never passed out before, but I have felt lightheaded and had similar symptoms like I was going to pass out.

Q: Are you always running or exercising when you feel these things?

A: Yes. It's usually when my heart rate gets really high, like 180 to 190 beats per minute.

Q: **Do you know what your normal resting heart rate is?**

A: Around 50 to 60 beats per minute.

Q: **Have you traveled anywhere recently?**

A: No.

Both providers asked important details about the symptoms and activities surrounding her event. They both asked about loss of bladder or bowel control, which can occur often in the setting of seizures (Asadi-Pooya, Emami, & Emami, 2014). The emergency department provider asked if the patient had ever had an episode in which she passed out, and she answered no. But she did not elaborate on the fact she had felt near-syncopal on previous occasions. The cardiovascular clinician was able to extract that information by being more specific in the questioning. In addition, the patient was asked about not only lightheadedness, but about any other symptoms she felt leading up to the event.

This information defines the character, but also associated symptoms, and, as we have seen in previous chapters, the questions often overlap to sometimes encompass more than one key feature at a time. The character of syncope is hard to define, and it is really the supporting and surrounding symptoms that help identify the nature of the event. The second provider also asked about recent travel in an attempt to identify any other diagnoses that can cause syncope, such as venous thromboembolism, which can occur after periods of immobility during extended travel (Crous-Bou, Harrigton, & Kabrhel, 2016).

## Timing and Duration

The emergency physician asked the following questions about the timing and duration of the patient's syncopal event:

Q: **What time did this happen today?**

A: Around 2 p.m.

Q: **How long were you running prior to this event?**

A: I ran 3 miles, so about 30 minutes.

Q: At what point during your run or after did this event occur?

A: About 30 minutes after I had finished my run.

Q: How long were you unconscious for?

A: My husband said it was about a minute.

Q: Did you feel lightheaded when you woke up or would you say you were back to baseline?

A: I felt okay—back to my baseline.

The cardiovascular clinician asked the following questions regarding the timing and duration of the episode of syncope:

Q: What time did this happen today?

A: Around 2 p.m.

Q: How long were you running before you experienced symptoms of lightheadedness, palpitations, and chest tightness?

A: I was nearly done with my 3-mile run when I started to feel bad—so about 25 minutes.

Q: When did this event occur in relation to your run?

A: About 30 minutes after I had stopped running.

Q: You had said you felt these symptoms before when your heart rate is elevated. Do you know what your heart rate was during your run today?

A: I noticed my heart rate monitor got to 180, and then it stopped reading it.

Q: Were you aware of what your heart rate was once you stopped running?

A: No. I had stopped my monitor when I finished. But in the past, it has taken my heart rate a long time to come back to normal.

Q: When you say "a long time," what do you mean—minutes? Hours?

A: Sometimes I can feel my palpitations for up to an hour, depending on my exercise.

Q: **How long ago did you first notice these symptoms?**

A: I guess when I started running—which is about a month ago.

Q: **Have you ever had any palpitations or dizziness when you were younger, while playing or in sports?**

A: I was never very active as a kid. I don't recall ever feeling anything like this until recently.

Q: **How long were you unconscious?**

A: My husband says for a minute, maybe less.

Q: **Did you have continued symptoms when you woke up or were they resolved?**

A: I felt okay. I did not have any palpitations when I came to.

Q: **How do you feel right now? Any lightheadedness or palpitations?**

A: No.

The emergency department provider and the cardiovascular clinician both asked when the event occurred in relation to the patient's running, and they both asked how long it lasted. The cardiovascular clinician asked more details about similar symptoms the patient had experienced prior to the event, and the timing of such. Remember, the question we are trying to answer is whether the syncopal event was due to symptomatic bradycardia because of the current pulse rate and ECG.

The symptoms ceased once the episode of syncope had passed. The patient did not feel them after the event and, most importantly, is not experiencing them now despite the objective findings of a low heart rate. This is important to highlight.

## Associated Symptoms

The first provider did not ask about any associated symptoms, but asked only how the patient was feeling just before the event, which elicited the response of lightheadedness. The second provider asked the following questions in regard to associated symptoms:

**Q: Did you have any symptoms of lightheadedness, palpitations, dizziness, chest pain, tightness, or shortness of breath before passing out?**

A: I felt lightheaded and did have some palpitations just before I passed out.

**Q: Did you have these symptoms when you were running as well or did you feel any nausea or vomiting?**

A: I did feel some shortness of breath and chest tightness at the end of my run along with the palpitations and the feeling that I was going to pass out. I have had no nausea or vomiting.

**Q: Is there any other activity that you do in which you feel dizziness, or palpitations, or any of those other symptoms? For instance, eating, going to the bathroom, or heavy lifting?**

A: Now that you mention it, I do feel tired and sometimes get palpitations after eating a big meal. But not to the degree I feel when I exercise.

**Q: Are you ever dizzy when you get up from a lying to a standing position? Have you had any swelling, weight gain, or weight loss that has been unintentional?**

A: No, I'm not dizzy like that. I have no swelling and have lost weight intentionally over the past several months.

**Q: Any shortness of breath lying flat, or do you wake up at night gasping for air?**

A: No.

At this point we have identified that there is clearly an association between the patient's symptoms and exercise, and, to a lesser degree, eating. The cardiovascular clinician was able to identify that not only did the patient have a constellation of symptoms leading up to her syncopal episode, she has had these same symptoms previously but never lost consciousness.

Interestingly, the patient does not recall ever having these kinds of symptoms before she began running on a consistent basis. With a chief complaint of syncope, a timeline as well as any symptoms leading up to the event are imperative in making the right diagnosis.

## Mitigating or Alleviating Factors

In this clinical scenario, neither provider asked questions directly related to mitigating or alleviating factors; however, it was evident during both evaluations that running or exercise seemed to elicit symptoms that ultimately resulted in an episode of syncope. The cardiovascular clinician asked the following:

> Q: **When you have felt these symptoms in the past, does anything make them better?**
>
> A: Usually once I stop running and rest for a while, I feel better. I have tried to drink more water thinking I was dehydrated, but it doesn't make much difference.
>
> Q: **You stated you get milder symptoms with eating. Is it always with eating or only with large meals?**
>
> A: It seems to be with large meals.

Syncope can be triggered by various things, depending on the causative mechanism. It is important to determine the setting, events leading up to the syncopal episode, and any pattern of activity associated with similar symptoms. Treatment of symptoms that the patient perceives as near-syncopal can help determine a cause as well. For instance, the patient felt perhaps she was getting dehydrated, yet increasing her fluid intake did not alleviate the symptoms. Likewise, position changes did not trigger these symptoms as might have been expected with orthostatic syncope. Although often no clear diagnosis is made when patients present with syncope, these clues help narrow the differential list to come closer to determining a cause.

# KEY FEATURES OF THE DATA

As we have discussed in previous chapters, the key features of the data include the available objective information we have so far as well as medications and relevant histories. When a patient presents with syncope, disturbances in electrolytes and any abnormal vital signs are crucial. In addition, ECGs are helpful to identify any rhythm abnormalities. Let us break down the data further.

## Vital Signs

The following findings were reported:

*Blood pressure*: 123/54 mmHg

*Pulse*: 45 beats per minute

*Respirations*: 14 breaths per minute

*Oxygen saturation*: 98% on room air

*Temperature*: 37.0°C

Blood pressures were repeated in both arms and were as follows:

*Left*: 126/65 mmHg

*Right*: 124/60 mmHg

Orthostatic blood pressure and pulse were assessed and were as follows:

*Lying*: 126/66 mmHg; pulse, 46 beats per minute

*Sitting*: 124/64 mmHg; pulse, 45 beats per minute

*Standing*: 126/60 mmHg; pulse, 48 beats per minute.

The patient does not have evidence of orthostatic hypotension; however, she is bradycardic.

## Electrocardiogram (ECG)

The initial ECG demonstrated bradycardia with premature ventricular contractions (PVCs) in a pattern of bigeminy. Bigeminy can cause near-syncope or syncope because it essentially halves the normal pulse rate, thereby reducing cardiac output (Keany, 2017). There was no evidence of ST or T-wave abnormalities to suggest ischemia. The voltage was normal. The QRS complex was narrow and QTc was within normal limits. When evaluating a patient with syncope, it is important to carefully review the ECG not only for arrhythmias, but for QT prolongation as this can precipitate ventricular arrhythmias and syncope (Wilde et al., 2016).

The presence of ventricular bigeminy in normal, healthy individuals usually does not require treatment unless associated symptoms are present; however, increased frequency of premature beats or four or more PVCs in a row (classified as ventricular tachycardia [VT]) can be problematic and should be cause for concern (Olgin & Zipes, 2015).

## Chest Radiograph

The chest film did not show any signs of pulmonary edema, infection, or lung abnormality. Heart size was within normal limits. There was no widening of the mediastinum.

## Biomarkers and Lab Results

The causes of syncope are numerous. It is important to review the laboratory data to exclude electrolyte abnormalities, anemia, infection, and myocardial infarction as potential reasons for the patient's symptoms. In this case the laboratory data were completely unremarkable, without any abnormalities that would warrant further evaluation.

## Other Data

The patient's medications were reviewed. She is not on any prescription medications. She takes a daily multivitamin, calcium supplements, and vitamin D and $B_{12}$. Her only medical history is uterine fibroids and recurrent ovarian cysts for which she mentioned she had a total hysterectomy. The cardiovascular clinician clarifies that she also had a bilateral salpingo-oophorectomy.

The patient is not on hormone replacement therapy and has lost 15 pounds since her surgery with diet and regular exercise. She is a life-long nonsmoker and drinks on occasion. She is adopted and is unaware of her biological parents' family history. She has no siblings and no children but is married. She does not use energy drinks, nutritional supplements, or weight loss supplements.

# DIFFERENTIALS AND DIFFERENCES IN EXAM

The three different categories of syncope should be considered during the evaluation and especially the examination of a patient who presents with this chief complaint. Subtle but characteristic features that can be found on the clinical exam can help classify the type of syncope the patient experienced.

Cardiovascular clinicians typically develop a regimented approach to the physical exam over time that is consistent for each patient evaluated. However, variations may occur when the clinician has a specific diagnosis in mind and is trying to confirm or rule it out. In a patient with syncope, the neurological portion of the exam can be just as important as the cardiovascular exam.

The patient's exam results, as noted by the emergency physician, were unremarkable. The cardiovascular clinician practitioner examines the patient and notes the following findings:

*General appearance: Well-nourished, well-developed White female in no acute distress.*

*Head and neck: Head is normocephalic and atraumatic, without lesions or masses. Neck is soft and supple, without thyromegaly or lymphadenopathy. Sclera are anicteric. Mucous membranes are moist. No intraoral lesions noted.*

*Cardiac exam: There is no elevation of jugular venous pressure. Peripheral pulses are palpable and symmetric. Carotid pulse is brisk bilaterally without bruits. No abdominal or femoral bruits. Auscultation of the heart revealed a bradycardic, regular rhythm. S1 and S2 present. No S3 or S4. No murmurs at rest, however I/VI systolic murmur noted with Valsalva and augmented in Valsalva post-extrasystole beat, best heard at the left sternal border. Diminished carotid pulse noted on post-extrasystole beat as well. Apical impulse is bounding but nondisplaced. Chest wall is nontender to palpation.*

*Lungs: Clear breath sounds throughout all lung fields with symmetric expansion.*

*Abdomen: Soft, nontender. Bowel sounds present in all four quadrants. No hepatosplenomegaly. No hepatojugular reflux.*

*Extremities: Warm, dry. No edema, clubbing, or cyanosis.*

*Neurological: Alert and oriented × 3. Cranial nerves are intact. Motor strength is symmetric in bilateral upper and lower extremities. No focal neurological deficits noted.*

The patient has now been evaluated thoroughly by both providers. The cardiovascular clinician is able to gain more insight into the patient's presenting complaint that establishes a pattern and association with exercise. This was not clearly identified by the first provider.

In addition, the cardiovascular clinician notes the physical exam finding of a murmur present only with Valsalva and the change in pulse on the post-PVC beat. The first provider did not pick up on this finding because it was not present at rest and there were no maneuvers done to elicit this change.

Based on the patient's history and the physical exam findings observed by the cardiovascular clinician, symptomatic bradycardia is unlikely to be the cause of this patient's syncope. What do you think is the most likely diagnosis?

There are many possible differential diagnoses for syncope. The list is probably more extensive than any other chief complaint we discuss in this book. As mentioned earlier, syncope can range from benign to life threatening. With that in mind, we will focus on the more common and the more serious or potentially life-threatening causes of syncope in our differential diagnosis list.

### Differential Diagnoses of Syncope

- Acute aortic dissection
- Aortic stenosis
- Bradyarrhythmias
- Brugada syndrome
- Cardiac tamponade
- Coronary artery disease/ischemia

- HCM
- Myocardial infarction
- Orthostatic syncope
- PAH
- Pulmonary embolus
- Seizure/epilepsy

- Severe anemia
- Tachyarrhythmias
- TIA
- Vasovagal syncope

HCM, hypertrophic cardiomyopathy; PAH, pulmonary arterial hypertension; TIA, transient ischemic attack.

## PULLING IT ALL TOGETHER

### Working Through the Differential

We can eliminate transient ischemic attack (TIA), seizure, and severe anemia right away in this patient. Although loss of consciousness can occur in both seizures and TIAs, these events do not produce true syncope because they do not result from reduction in cerebral blood flow (as occurs with syncope). In a TIA there has to be some associated neurological deficit associated with the loss of consciousness. Neither seizures nor TIAs result in spontaneous recovery with immediate return to baseline condition (Calkins & Zipes, 2015), which is characteristic of syncope. Severe anemia is also easily eliminated based on the patient's normal complete blood count (CBC). To summarize, TIA, seizure, and anemia can be ruled out based on the following:

- No associated neurological deficit
- No seizure-like activity (tongue biting, tonic–clonic movement, or incontinence)
- Rapid recovery to baseline
- Normal hemoglobin and hematocrit on CBC

The most common causes of syncope are vasovagal syncope and orthostatic syncope (Sutton, 2013). Vasovagal syncope falls under the category of reflex-mediated syncope and is also known as "neurally mediated syncope." It is usually caused by a sudden drop in heart rate and blood pressure and can be triggered from a situational event such as coughing, voiding, or weight lifting, to name a few (Sutton, 2013).

It this patient's case, we do not know her blood pressure during the event or leading up to it. She reports that her heart rate was fast when she began to have symptoms. These symptoms were present in similar situations, so vasovagal syncope is still a possibility, but not at the top of our list. Orthostatic syncope can include volume depletion, drug effects, and autonomic failure. We can reasonably eliminate this from our differential based on the following:

- No signs of dehydration or volume depletion; patient reports increased hydration with exercise, as well
- Not orthostatic based on blood pressure/heart rate findings
- No drugs taken to precipitate drop in blood pressure or cause for syncope

Acute aortic dissection can present as syncope, particularly if there is cardiac tamponade; however, in those cases patients are usually in acute distress and potentially in cardiogenic shock. So, we are probably safe to eliminate this based on the following:

- No back or chest pain currently
- Symmetric blood pressures
- No widening of the mediastinum on chest film
- Hemodynamically stable

Syncope and sudden cardiac death have been known to occur in patients with pulmonary arterial hypertension (PAH; Mar et al., 2015). According to Mar and colleagues (2015), the Valsalva maneuver contributed to increased risk of syncope in patients with pulmonary hypertension, as well. Most of the patients in this study already had a diagnosis of PAH and were on drug therapy that lowered systemic blood pressure—which can also contribute to syncope. Further diagnostic evaluation, such as an echocardiogram or coronary angiography, is needed to completely eliminate this diagnosis as a possible cause of syncope in this patient's case.

What about pulmonary embolus? Syncope can occur when there is sudden obstruction of the most proximal pulmonary arteries or a significant obstruction to cause reduction in cardiac output (Prandoni et al., 2016). However, other features are often present with pulmonary embolus—features this patient did not have. We can eliminate this diagnosis simply based on the following:

- Negative D-dimer
- No shortness of breath or tachypnea
- No tachycardia
- No hypoxia

Syncope in the absence of any ECG changes suggestive of ischemia or symptoms suggestive of angina is unlikely to be caused by myocardial infarction. This patient did have chest tightness associated with shortness of breath and high heart rates, so one could suggest these were anginal symptoms. In addition, bradyarrhythmias can be present in the setting of an inferior myocardial infarction due to the location of the right coronary artery and the atrioventricular (AV) node (Goldstein, Lee, Pica, Dixon, & O'Neill, 2005). However, her symptoms correlated with high heart rates, not bigeminy or bradycardia.

Her ECG did not demonstrate signs of ischemia or infarction, and her troponin T level was undetectable nearly 3 hours after the event. We can reasonably rule out myocardial infarction; however, we cannot necessarily rule out the presence of coronary artery disease or ischemia at this point. Severe ischemia, however, does not typically cause the depressed cardiac output required to cause syncope (Mitrani & Hendel, 2013). It is more likely for ischemia to produce an arrhythmia, and that is the mechanism which results in syncope. So myocardial ischemia cannot be entirely eliminated as a cause, but it is lower on the differential list based on the following:

- No ECG findings suggestive of ischemia or infarction
- No cardiac risk factors for coronary artery disease
- Negative troponin

The clinical picture of syncope in this case is not consistent with a diagnosis of cardiac tamponade. We can eliminate this from our list for the following reasons:

- Cardiac silhouette normal on chest film
- Hemodynamically stable and not in distress
- No jugular venous distension
- No bedside pulsus paradoxus

Brugada syndrome is an inherited condition characterized by coved ST-segment elevation in the right precordial leads and an incomplete right bundle branch block. It is associated with ventricular arrhythmias and sudden cardiac death (Sieira et al., 2016). This patient's ECG did not show any abnormalities suggestive of this condition; therefore, we can eliminate it as a possibility.

Aortic stenosis can cause obstruction of the left ventricular outflow tract (LVOT) due to narrowing of the aortic valve opening. Syncope can be a manifestation of this obstruction, due to decreased cardiac output or at times of decreased preload, but typically it does not occur until later stages of the disease (Cary & Pearce, 2013). Patients with aortic stenosis typically have a crescendo-decrescendo pattern systolic murmur present at rest that decreases in intensity during the Valsalva maneuver. Our patient had no murmur at rest; however, with Valsalva maneuver a slight murmur was noted. Often patients with aortic stenosis have symptoms of heart failure as well, and this patient does not. An echocardiogram is the gold standard to confirm this diagnosis, but based on her presentation and clinical exam findings, this can be moved lower on our differential list.

What about the possibility of any tachy- or bradyarrhythmias? The initial thought was that this patient had syncope due to symptomatic bradycardia and the presence of bigeminy. The patient stated her normal resting heart rate is between 50 and 60 beats per minute. Her heart rate on evaluation was 45 beats per minute and bigeminy was noted, which as Keany (2017) noted can cause syncope since the rate is essentially halved by the premature ventricular beats. If she had symptoms of lightheadedness, dizziness, or signs of decreased perfusion, this might be the right diagnosis. But based on the following findings, it is less likely:

- No signs of decreased perfusion, as evidenced by good mentation and normal blood pressure
- No symptoms of lightheadedness or near syncope with present heart rate
- Baseline heart rate not much higher than current heart rate
- Symptoms preceding syncopal event correlated with high heart rates, not low

So, is it possible that the patient is having a tachyarrhythmia, such as supraventricular tachycardia (SVT), or bursts of VT? According to the American Heart Association (2017, March 21), the calculated maximum heart rate for a patient of 47 years is 173 beats per minute (220 minus the patient's age). She was reaching much higher rates of 180 to 190 beats per minute. We do not know whether sinus tachycardia or something more sinister caused her symptoms. It is quite possible she was having symptoms and a subsequent syncopal spell due to the rapid heart rate. This possibility is higher on our differential list at this point based on the preceding information.

Lastly, we have hypertrophic cardiomyopathy (HCM). Several important features of this disease can be found in the patient's history as well as the physical exam. Let us review the highlights, as outlined by Maron and Olivotto (2015), to see if our patient has any findings that are consistent with this diagnosis.

- HCM can be obstructive or nonobstructive. Patients with the nonobstructive form develop latent obstruction with exercise.
- HCM can be hereditary. There is often a family history of syncope or sudden cardiac death.
- A murmur can be absent at rest, and it increases with the Valsalva maneuver (in contrast to aortic stenosis, where the opposite occurs).
- Pulse pressure decreases on the post-PVC beat (the opposite occurs in aortic stenosis).
- Women can be underdiagnosed and often are diagnosed at later ages.
- Patients can have bradycardia, syncope, and VT.
- The ECG can be normal or show increased voltages consistent with left ventricular hypertrophy or ST/T-wave changes.

Now let us review the highlights of our patient's case:

- Unsure of family history (adopted)
- Normal ECG
- No murmur at rest, but present with Valsalva
- Diminished pulse post-PVC beat with increased murmur
- Syncope, and near syncope with elevated heart rates, primarily during exercise

Do you think this patient had syncope due to a primary diagnosis of HCM? This is the most likely diagnosis based on all the data and, in particular, her physical exam findings. She may have had VT that precipitated her syncope, but the VT may have been caused by the underlying HCM and the occurrence of LVOT obstruction during exercise, so her diagnosis of syncope may be twofold.

The presence of PVCs and the diminished pulse pressure with the post-PVC beat is a key clinical feature of HCM, referred to as the Brockenbrough–Braunwald–Morrow sign (Trevino & Buergler, 2014). If she had had a positive family history of syncope, this would further support the diagnosis, as it is an inherited disorder. However, she was adopted and has no knowledge of her biological family's medical history.

It is important to point out that this patient only recently began to exercise actively, which might explain the absence of symptoms up until now. She also had symptoms after eating a large meal, which can occur in HCM (Adams et al., 2015). Syncope in patients with HCM often occurs 30 minutes to an hour after exercise (Maron & Olivotto, 2015), as occurred in this case. In addition, the patient had had a total hysterectomy with bilateral salpingo-oophorectomy, likely causing early menopause, and is not on any hormone replacement therapy. Research has suggested a possible link to estrogen in delaying hypertrophy (Pedram et al, 2013). This might explain why women tend to be diagnosed with HCM later in life, after menopause. Further studies are needed, however, to prove a direct link.

**Likely Diagnosis:** HCM

---

## WHAT'S NEXT?

- *The patient is admitted to the hospital for further evaluation.*
- An echocardiogram shows asymmetric septal hypertrophy with a septal thickness measuring 16 mm. The ejection fraction is preserved at 65%, and there are no valvular abnormalities and no PAH.
- An exercise stress test demonstrates dynamic LVOT obstruction following exercise with a gradient as high as 50 mmHg. The patient becomes hypotensive after peak exercise and develops symptoms similar to her presentation. ST depression is also noted with exertion and a 6-beat run of nonsustained VT.
- Coronary angiography reveals no obstructive disease.
- She is started on low-dose beta-blocker therapy and undergoes placement of an implantable cardiac defibrillator based on guideline-directed therapy for the prevention of sudden cardiac death (Anastasakis et al., 2014).

---

# SUMMARIZING THE SCENARIO

Syncope can cause a diagnostic dilemma for many clinicians in the acute care setting. A detailed timeline of events leading up to and surrounding the episode of syncope are crucial in obtaining an accurate diagnosis. The emergency department provider asked appropriate and detailed questions about the actual event and symptoms preceding the syncope. The cardiovascular clinician was able to extract more details about the symptoms associated with the event and symptoms experienced prior to the event through comprehensive questioning. This established a time-line and clear pattern of exercise-induced symptoms.

Initially the diagnosis was thought to be symptomatic bradycardia in the setting of bigeminy and a low heart rate. However, obtaining a more detailed history, including an account of baseline heart rate as well as current symptoms, negated this thought process. Other factors, such as age, prior history, and medications, were also considered, helping to eliminate additional diagnoses.

The exam performed by the first provider did not reveal any abnormalities, but the cardiovascular clinician had already considered HCM as a probable diagnosis given the history and assessed for any changes with Valsalva maneuver and post-extrasystole beats. The additional information obtained further supported the cardiovascular clinician's suspicion, leading to the most likely diagnosis of HCM and possible VT as the cause of the syncopal episode. This diagnosis was confirmed by echocardiography.

Without a detailed assessment of symptoms, associated symptoms, and activity surrounding syncope, the right diagnosis can be missed. In many cases a diagnosis is not made until several episodes of syncope have occurred. It was beneficial in this case that the patient's husband was able to witness the event and give further insight about what transpired during the time that she was unconscious. Without this information, it might have been harder to differentiate between true syncope and a seizure.

The diagnosis of HCM is not one that is frequently made in the emergency department setting. The emergency physician did a thorough assessment and evaluation, but the cardiovascular clinician's input was invaluable because of that provider's experience and knowledge of this often-elusive condition.

In Chapter 6, we look at another example of syncope by way of a somewhat different interaction between a patient and healthcare providers.

# REFERENCES

Adams, J., Bois, J., Masaki, M., Yuasa, T., Oh, J., Ommen, S., ... Klarich, K. (2015). Postprandial hemodynamics in hypertrophic cardiomyopathy. *Echocardiography, 32*(11), 1614–1620.

American Heart Association. (2017, March 21). Target heart rates. Retrieved from http://www.heart.org/HEARTORG/HealthyLiving/PhysicalActivity/FitnessBasics/Target-Heart-Rates_UCM_434341_Article.jsp#WNE_KYWcGM8

Anastasakis, A., Borger, M., Borggrete, M., Cecchi, C., Charron, P., Hagege, A., ... Sekhri, N. (2014). 2014 ESC Guidelines on diagnosis and management of hypertrophic cardiomyopathy: The Task Force for the Diagnosis and Management of Hypertrophic Cardiomyopathy of the European Society of Cardiology (ESC). *European Heart Journal, 35*(39). 2733–2779.

Asadi-Pooya, A., Emami, M., & Emami, Y. (2014). Ictal injury in psychogenic non-epileptic seizures. *Seizure, 23*(5), 363–366. doi:10.1016/j.seizure.2014.03.001

Calkins, H., & Zipes, D. (2015). Hypotension and syncope. In *Braunwald's heart disease: A textbook of cardiovascular medicine* (10th ed.). Philadelphia, PA: Elsevier/Saunders.

Cary, T., & Pearce, J. (2013). Aortic stenosis: Pathophysiology, diagnosis, and medical management of non-surgical patients. *Critical Care Nurse, 33*(2), 58–72. doi:10.4037/ccn2013820

Crous-Bou, M., Harrington, L., & Kabrhel, C. (2016). Environmental and genetic risk factors associated with venous thromboembolism. *Seminars in Thrombosis and Hemostatis, 42*(8), 808–820.

Farlex Partner Medical Dictionary. (2012). Syncope. Retrieved from http://medical-dictionary.thefreedictionary.com/syncope

Goldstein, J., Lee, D., Pica, M., Dixon, S., & O'Neill, W. (2005). Patterns of coronary compromise leading to bradyarrhythmias and hypotension in inferior myocardial infarction. *Coronary Artery Disease, 16*(5), 264–274.

Guzman, J., & Morillo, C. (2015). Syncope and driving. *Cardiology Clinics, 33*(3), 465–471.

Keany, J. (2017). Premature ventricular contraction clinical presentation. Retrieved from http://emedicine.medscape.com/article/761148-clinical

Mar, P., Nwazue, V., Black, B., Biaggioni, I., Deidrich, A., Oaranjape, S., ... Hemnes, A. (2016). Valsalva maneuver in pulmonary arterial hypertension: Susceptibility to syncope and autonomic dysfunction. *Chest, 149*(5), 1252–1260. doi:10.1016/j.chest.2015.11.015

Maron, B., & Olivotto, I. (2015). Hypertrophic cardiomyopathy. In D. L. Mann, D. P. Zipes, P. Libby, & R. O. Bonow, *Braunwald's heart disease: A textbook of cardiovascular medicine* (10th ed., pp. 1574–1588). Philadelphia, PA: Elsevier/ Saunders.

Mitrani, R., & Hendel, R. (2013). The appropriateness of an ischemic evaluation for syncope. *Circulation, 6*(3), 358–359. doi:10.1161.CIRCIMAGING.113.000301

Olgin, J., & Zipes, D. (2015). Specific arrhythmias: Diagnosis and treatment. In *Braunwald's heart disease: A textbook of cardiovascular medicine* (10th ed.). Philadelphia, PA: Elsevier/Saunders.

Patel, P., & Quinn, J. (2015). Syncope: A review of emergency department management and disposition. *Clinical and Experimental Emergency Medicine, 2*(2), 67–74.

Pedram, A., Razandi, M., Narayanan, R., Dalton, J., McKinsey, T., & Levin, E. (2013). Estrogen regulates histone deacetylases to prevent cardiac hypertrophy. *Molecular Biology of the Cell, 24*(24), 3805–3818.

Prandoni, P., Anthonie, W., Lensing, M., Prins, M., Ciammaichella, M., Perlati, M., ... Barbar, S. (2016). Prevalence of pulmonary embolism among patients hospitalized for syncope. *The New England Journal of Medicine, 375,* 1524–1531. doi:10.1056/NEJMoa162172

Saklani, P., Krahn, A., & Klein, G. (2013). Syncope. *Circulation, 127,* 1330–1339.

Sieira, J., Conte, G., Ciconte, G., de Asmundis, C., Gian-Battista, C., Baltogiannis, G., ... Brugada, P. (2016). Clinical characterization and long-term prognosis of women with Brugada syndrome. *Heart, 102,* 452–458. doi:10.1136/ heartjnl-2015-308556

Sutton, B. (2013). Clinical classification of syncope. *Progress in Cardiovascular Disease, 55*(4), 339–344. doi:10.1016/j.pcad.2012.11.005

Trevino, A., & Buergler, J. (2014). The Brockenbrough-Braunwald-Morrow sign. *Methodist DeBakey Cardiovascular Journal, 10*(1), 34–37.

Wilde, A., Moss, A., Kaufman, E., Shimizu, W., Peterson, D., Benhorin, J., ... Ackerman, M. (2016). Clinical aspects of type 3 long-QT syndrome: An international multicenter study. *Circulation, 134*(12), 872–882. doi:10.10.1131/ CIRCULATIONAHA.116.021823

# CHAPTER 6

# Syncope: Another Encounter

In Chapter 5, the initial presentation for a patient with syncope was related and key features of the data obtained by the emergency physician and the cardiovascular clinician were extracted and compared. In this chapter, we review another interaction involving a patient with syncope, contrasting the details obtained by two providers evaluating the scenario from different perspectives. The initial interview process is described, and the histories obtained by each provider are summarized. Then the key features of the history are compared. By this point in the book, you should be better able to identify key features of the history and know how to obtain the data during the initial interaction.

## CASE SCENARIO

A 70-year-old obese White male is brought into the emergency department at 9:00 a.m. by EMS after experiencing an episode of syncope. An ECG obtained in the field shows atrial fibrillation with a rate of 115 beats per minute. The patient is hypotensive, with blood pressure of 95/62 mmHg. His oxygen saturation is 88%. He is afebrile.

EMS, emergency medical services.

The emergency department provider asks the following questions to obtain a history:

**Q: Can you tell me what happened today that prompted you to call emergency medical services (EMS)?**

A: I passed out.

**Q: What were you doing prior to this episode?**

A: I was cleaning up the table after breakfast, and I felt dizzy and lightheaded. Next thing I know I woke up and I was on the floor.

**Q: Did you injure anything or are you in pain?**

A: My shoulder is a little sore, but nothing else that I noticed.

**Q: What time did this occur?**

A: Around 8:00 a.m. I think.

**Q: Do you have any idea how long you were out?**

A: No, maybe a few minutes. I looked at the clock when I was eating breakfast at 7:45. It takes me about 10 to 15 minutes to eat. I had my phone in my pocket and called 911 when I woke up. It was 8:05 then.

**Q: How did you feel when you woke up? Still dizzy or lightheaded, or were you back to baseline?**

A: I felt okay. Not dizzy, just not right. My shoulder hurt and I wasn't sure what happened so I called an ambulance.

**Q: Do you live with anyone who witnessed this?**

A: No, I'm widowed. I live alone.

**Q: Did you lose control of your bladder or bowels?**

A: No.

**Q: Have you ever had an episode like this before where you lost consciousness?**

A: No.

**Q: Do you have any history of heart problems such as an abnormal heart rhythm, heart attack, or stroke?**

A: No. I have high blood pressure and high cholesterol.

**Q: How are you feeling right now?**

A: Not that great. I feel like I can't get a deep breath. I'm tired.

An ECG is repeated in the emergency department. It shows no signs of ischemia but does show atrial fibrillation with a rate of 110 beats per minute. A chest film does not show any acute process and the complete blood count (CBC) and chemistry panel results are within normal limits. A CT scan of the head is obtained, and findings are also normal. Shoulder and arm radiographs demonstrate only soft tissue injury and no fractures. The troponin T level is 0.10 ng/mL.

The emergency department provider performs a complete physical exam and notes the patient to be clammy and in a mild amount of distress, but the findings are otherwise unremarkable. The patient is placed on oxygen at 2 L/min via nasal cannula. A cardiology consultation is requested to evaluate this patient for new-onset atrial fibrillation and syncope. The emergency department provider summarizes the information for the cardiovascular clinician in history A.

# HISTORY A

*A 70-year-old obese White male with a history of hypertension and hyperlipidemia presents to the emergency department after experiencing an episode of syncope. He was cleaning up dishes from the table when he became lightheaded and dizzy. He woke up on the floor with pain in his shoulder from the fall but otherwise sustained no injuries. The event was unwitnessed, but he denies any loss of bladder or bowel function. He still feels poorly, reporting difficulty in taking a deep breath. Rescue arrived and ECG done at the scene demonstrated atrial fibrillation with a rate of 115 beats per minute. He remains in atrial fibrillation and is hypotensive and clammy. Imaging as well as laboratory data are unremarkable except for a troponin T level of 0.10 ng/mL. He is now on 2 L/min of oxygen via nasal cannula saturating at 90%. We are concerned his syncopal spell may be caused by his new arrhythmia or may be ischemia, based on the troponin level.*

What are your initial thoughts? Is there any piece of the history that is missing? What else do we need to know in order to make the right diagnosis quickly? Let us see what else the cardiology consultant is able to find out.

The cardiovascular clinician arrives at the patient's bedside and obtains the following vital signs: Blood pressure, 105/76 mmHg; pulse, 112 beats per minute, with atrial fibrillation noted on the telemetry monitor; respiratory rate, 24 breaths per minute; oxygen saturation, now 91% on 2 L/min of oxygen, which is increased to 4 L/min. The patient is afebrile.

The cardiovascular clinician asks the patient the following questions:

Q: **What happened today that brought you to the emergency department?**

A: I passed out.

Q: **Has this ever happened to you before?**

A: No.

Q: **What were you doing when this occurred?**

A: I had just finished breakfast and was clearing the table. I started to feel lightheaded and dizzy, and the next thing I knew I was on the floor.

Q: **Did you try to sit down or lie down when you felt this way prior to passing out?**

A: I was able to set the dishes down and I leaned over the counter.

Q: **Do you know what time it was when this happened?**

A: I started eating at 7:45. It usually takes me around 10 to 15 minutes. When I looked at my phone to call 911 it was 8:05.

Q: **Did you hurt yourself?**

A: I fell on my shoulder, I guess, because it's really sore, but nothing else.

Q: **How were you feeling this morning when you got up prior to the event? Were you having any chest discomfort, shortness of breath, palpations, nausea, sweatiness, or lightheadedness?**

A: Not really. I didn't feel great, but I can't really describe it. I feel like I can't get a deep breath.

Q: **Did you feel that sensation before you passed out? Or have you had these symptoms any time in the past?**

A: I may have felt the shortness of breath before, but I've never had anything like this until today.

Q: **Do you ever get dizzy or lightheaded when you go from a lying to standing position?**

A: No.

Q: **How did you feel last night?**

A: I felt normal. It was only this morning I noticed a change.

Q: **How did you feel when you came to? Any confusion or disorientation?**

A: My shoulder was hurting. I wasn't confused and I knew where I was, but I didn't feel right. I can't describe it. Just that something was wrong.

Q: **Are you aware of your rapid heartbeat now?**

A: No.

Q: **Are you having any chest pain, dizziness, or nausea now?**

A: No, but I don't feel good. I feel like something is really wrong.

Q: **Have you ever had any history of heart problems, such as an abnormal heartbeat, heart attack, heart failure, or stroke?**

A: No.

Q: **I see you have high blood pressure and high cholesterol. Are you diabetic or do you have any thyroid problems, history of cancer, or blood clots or bleeding disorders?**

A: No. I've been told I'm prediabetic. But I've started to diet and already lost 10 pounds this past month. I also walk 20 minutes a day. I have never had any blood clots and I haven't had any cancer or issues with bleeding.

Q: **Do you ever have shortness of breath, chest pain, or dizziness during your walks?**

A: No. I take it nice and slow, though.

Q: **Do you take medication for your high blood pressure and high cholesterol?**

A: Yes. I take lisinopril, 20 mg daily, and atorvastatin, 40 mg at night. I haven't taken any medication yet today.

**Q: Do you ever take your blood pressure or pulse at home? If so, do you recall the readings?**

A: I check it in those machines at the grocery store every once in a while. My blood pressure is usually 130s over 80s and my heart rate is in the 70s.

**Q: Do you see your primary care physician on a regular basis? Have you ever had any cardiac workup, such as a stress test or heart catheterization?**

A: I get my annual physicals. I had a stress test 2 years ago and it was fine.

**Q: Do you snore or have sleep apnea?**

A: My wife used to tell me I snore. I haven't been tested for sleep apnea.

**Q: Have you traveled anywhere recently?**

A: No.

**Q: Have you been sick recently or around anyone who has been sick?**

A: No.

**Q: Any recent surgeries?**

A: No.

**Q: Do you drink or smoke? Did you eat anything out of the ordinary in the past 24 hours?**

A: I don't drink at all. I smoked for about 5 years back in my 30s. I haven't eaten anything out of the ordinary.

**Q: Any family history of heart problems?**

A: Not that I'm aware of.

The cardiovascular clinician summarizes the information obtained from the patient in history B.

# HISTORY B

*A 70-year-old obese White male with a prior history of only hypertension and hyperlipidemia presented to the emergency department this morning around*

9 a.m. via EMS after having a syncopal event. He was clearing the dishes from the table when he began to feel lightheaded and dizzy, prompting him to lean over the counter. He awoke on the floor with pain in his shoulder from the fall but had no other injuries. He is unsure how long he was out, but based on the time he believes only minutes.

He reports feeling unwell this morning before the event but denies chest pain, palpitations, nausea, or vomiting. He feels like he is unable to take a deep breath currently and thinks he may have felt this prior to the event as well. He called 911 after this episode. He was hypotensive when EMS arrived, and an ECG at the time demonstrated atrial fibrillation, which remains present. Laboratory data are significant only for a troponin T level of 0.10 ng/mL.

He has no history of arrhythmias or coronary artery disease, heart failure, blood clots, stroke, or diabetes. He reported a normal stress test 2 years ago and follows up regularly with his primary care physician. He has been told he is prediabetic, and he recently started dieting and has lost 10 lb in the past month. He has never been diagnosed with sleep apnea but does admit to snoring. He denies any recent illness, travel, or sick contacts. He continues to feel generally unwell—stating "something is wrong," despite improvement in blood pressure and oxygen supplementation—but denies chest pain, dizziness, or lightheadedness.

Based on the preceding history, do you have any more insight as to what might have precipitated this patient's syncopal event?

# KEY FEATURES OF THE HISTORY

The information obtained by both providers provided details surrounding the event of syncope; however, the cardiovascular clinician asked more comprehensive questions about relevant past history and preceding symptoms. The initial thought was that the presence of atrial fibrillation and/or possibly ischemia caused the episode of syncope. What do you think? Let us review and compare the key features that each provider obtained.

## Character

Both providers asked the patient what he was doing and what symptoms he felt right before the event. They both inquired whether any injuries were sustained and whether he had ever had an episode like this in the past. They also identified how the patient was currently feeling.

The cardiovascular clinician asked detailed questions about how the patient was feeling earlier in the morning in order to assess whether the symptoms were abrupt, or whether he had not been feeling well in the hours leading up to the event. The patient was asked about symptoms consistent with orthostasis, which he denied.

He was also asked about recent illnesses or travel, which are important questions when trying to identify factors that might have led up to the event. Both providers asked about incontinence to exclude seizure as a possibility, but the cardiovascular clinician went on to ask about the patient's mental state after he came around to further identify whether this loss of consciousness was related to a neurological event. Each piece of information helps to narrow the possible causes.

We know that the patient has atrial fibrillation, which is a new diagnosis for him, and that he was also more hypotensive initially. Asking about baseline heart rate and any symptoms presently being experienced helps identify whether there is an association between the arrhythmia, the low blood pressure, and the loss of consciousness.

## Timing and Duration

Each provider asked when the event happened and approximately how long it lasted. In this case, there were no witnesses to give an exact account, but luckily the patient was able to recall what time it was prior to and shortly after he lost consciousness, which helped to determine that the episode likely lasted a few minutes at most. The patient also told both clinicians that he began to feel lightheaded and dizzy just before he passed out but did not have these feelings for any length of time leading up to the event.

His account of the episode suggests that he had complete recovery when he awoke other than the pain he felt from falling and the general feeling of unease that he had been experiencing throughout the morning. The cardiovascular clinician was also able to determine that the patient felt at his baseline the night before, which further establishes a timeline of events.

## Associated Symptoms

The emergency department provider asked the patient what he was feeling just before the event but did not ask about any other symptoms, such as chest discomfort, palpitations, nausea, or vomiting. The cardiology clinician asked about the presence of each of these symptoms specifically before, during, and after the event. The patient noted that he felt like he was unable to get a deep breath and mentions that he is still feeling this way.

When evaluating patients who have had syncope, all factors surrounding the event need to be taken into account. In orthostatic syncope, symptoms often occur with standing, and with vasovagal syncope, symptoms can include nausea, diaphoresis, and lightheadedness (Patel & Quinn, 2015). The patient experienced symptoms shortly after standing as he was clearing the table, so we can consider that perhaps he was orthostatic—especially given his blood pressure at first evaluation. However, he did not have any diaphoresis or nausea prior to the event. No other associated symptoms were identified.

## Mitigating or Alleviating Factors

This was the patient's first episode of syncope. Both providers were able to identify that. The cardiovascular clinician went on to ask whether the patient had had any similar symptoms before today. If he had, further questions about how those symptoms were brought on or alleviated might have helped in determining a cause. The only mitigating factor in this case is that the patient was clearing the table and had onset of symptoms. As mentioned before, it is possible the change in position from sitting to standing may have precipitated orthostasis and caused syncope but we cannot be sure.

The patient did try to alleviate the symptoms by leaning over the counter—which was discovered during the questioning by the cardiology consultant—but this did not help. Once the episode of syncope happened, the symptom of lightheadedness was alleviated.

If the patient felt well just up to the event and felt well after, we might be reassured; however, he has continued to feel poorly, suggesting something more sinister might have caused the event and might be ongoing.

# KEY FEATURES OF THE DATA

The key features of the data for this patient with syncope are the same as those listed for the patient discussed in Chapter 5. Once again it is important to examine any vital signs, laboratory data, imaging, medications, and other histories that might help us decipher the differential. Let us review the available data thus far and discuss their implications.

## Vital Signs

The following findings were reported:

*Blood pressure:* 105/76 mmHg

*Pulse:* 112 beats per minute

*Respirations:* 24 breaths per minute

*Oxygen saturation:* 93% on 4 L/min nasal cannula

*Temperature:* 37.1°C

The patient was initially more hypotensive when evaluated by EMS at the scene, with a blood pressure of 95/62 mmHg and a heart rate of 115 beats per minute. He is obese, and his body mass index is calculated at 41 kg/m². The cardiovascular clinician obtains repeat blood pressures on both arms, as follows:

*Right:* 102/74 mmHg

*Left:* 106/70 mmHg

Orthostatic vital signs are also obtained, as follows:

*Lying:* 108/72 mmHg

*Sitting:* 106/72 mmHg

*Standing:* 104/74 mmHg

The patient's heart rate remains between 109 and 115 beats per minute. He is tachypneic, and it is noteworthy that his oxygen saturation is only 93% despite oxygen supplementation.

## Electrocardiogram (ECG)

The initial ECG shows atrial fibrillation. The QRS is narrow. The QTc interval is normal. T-wave inversion is noted in leads V1 through V4.

No previous ECGs are available for comparison, but we do know that this is the first incidence of atrial fibrillation of which the patient is aware.

## Chest Radiograph

The chest film did not show any signs of infection, effusions, or pulmonary edema. There was no atelectasis or pneumothorax. There was mild cardiomegaly, but otherwise the study was normal. There are no other chest films with which to compare so we are unsure whether this cardiomegaly is new or old.

## Biomarkers and Lab Results

When a patient presents with syncope, looking for any electrolyte abnormalities is essential. This patient had a normal CBC and a normal chemistry panel. His glucose level was 122 mg/dL. The troponin T level, however, was abnormal at 0.10 ng/mL. As demonstrated in earlier chapters, however, troponin levels can be abnormal in conditions other than cardiac ischemia.

It is important to consider the context of the clinical presentation when interpreting the significance of the troponin result. Cardiac ischemia must be the first consideration, but in this case do you think that is the cause? A literature review reveals that patients with atrial fibrillation can have falsely elevated troponin levels (Parwani et al., 2013). The heart rate and symptoms of myocardial ischemia in these patients correlate to the abnormal level.

This patient's heart rate was elevated, but not extremely so, which should cause some speculation that this troponin level is truly a consequence of a high heart rate. He has risk factors for coronary artery disease, including obesity, hypertension, and hyperlipidemia. Is it possible his shortness of breath is an angina equivalent? Are there any other laboratory data you would want to review in this scenario that have not already been obtained?

What about a D-dimer level? The cardiovascular clinician added this test to the lab evaluation, and the result reported was 5.6 mcg/mL fibrinogen equivalent units (FEU), which is well above the normal level (<0.50 mcg/mL FEU). The D-dimer level can be elevated in various situations, including acute coronary syndromes, aortic dissections, and acute pulmonary embolisms (Pathak, Rendon, & Muthyala, 2011). This information is very helpful and should immediately cause you to narrow your working diagnosis.

## Other Data

The patient had a CT scan of the head as well as shoulder imaging to rule out any injuries or head trauma. Both studies were negative and showed only a soft tissue injury to his left shoulder. He was asked about medications and compliance by the cardiovascular clinician. He takes lisinopril, 20 mg daily, and atorvastatin, 40 mg every night. He has taken no medications today. He is obese and gives a history of hypertension and hyperlipidemia, which are both being treated based on his medications. He is prediabetic and mentions that he has recently started dieting and walking and has lost 10 pounds within the past month. He does not drink and he smoked for a brief period of time during his 30s. He has no surgical history.

He has no family history of heart disease or syncope. He has never had any history of heart problems or any other medical conditions not previously mentioned. He is followed regularly by his primary care physician and mentions having had a stress test within the past 2 years, results of which were normal. The cardiovascular clinician asked him why the stress test was done, and he stated it was for routine screening and not for any symptoms.

He was questioned about the presence of sleep apnea given his obesity and denied having a diagnosis, although he admits to snoring. This line of questioning is relevant because sleep apnea and hypertension are known triggers of atrial fibrillation. The cardiovascular clinician was trying to identify underlying risk factors that might predispose him to atrial fibrillation.

# DIFFERENTIALS AND DIFFERENCES IN EXAM

We discussed the three different categories of syncope in Chapter 5. Recall that these were reflex, orthostatic, and cardiac syncope. Considerations in evaluating this patient are the same as those in the Chapter 5 case.

The physical exam may be normal, or it may reveal minor abnormalities that might seem insignificant in another clinical context. This patient not only had syncope, he also has an arrhythmia. Therefore, the exam should focus on identifying any evidence that may help to determine the nature of both, or whether there is a relationship at all.

The cardiovascular clinician examines the patient and reports the following findings:

*General appearance: Well-nourished, pale, obese White male in a moderate amount of distress.*

*Head and neck: Head is normocephalic and atraumatic, without evidence of lesions or masses. Sclera are anicteric. Neck is soft and supple, without thyromegaly or lymphadenopathy.*

*Cardiac exam: No elevation of jugular venous pressure although exam is limited by body habitus. No carotid bruits. No femoral or abdominal bruits. Carotid upstrokes are symmetric and brisk. Peripheral pulses are palpable and symmetric. Auscultation of the heart reveals an irregularly irregular rhythm. S1 and S2 present, no S3 or S4. Mild right ventricular (RV) lift. No murmurs or rubs. Chest wall is nontender to palpation.*

*Lungs: Clear breath sounds in bilateral lung fields, slightly reduced bilaterally in bases—although patient has poor inspiratory effort, with tachypnea noted.*

*Abdomen: Obese. Nontender. Bowel sounds present in all four quadrants. No hepatosplenomegaly. No hepatojugular reflux.*

*Extremities: Slightly cool, dry. No edema. Ecchymosis and swelling noted on left shoulder, with associated tenderness.*

*Neurological: Alert and oriented × 3. Cranial nerves are intact. Motor strength is symmetric in bilateral upper and lower extremities. No focal neurological deficits.*

The patient has now been evaluated by both the emergency department provider and the cardiovascular clinician. A comprehensive history and physical exam have been completed, and all the available data reviewed. What do you think caused this patient's syncope? Do you think it is ischemia, arrhythmia, or something else? Based on the D-dimer level and his symptoms, you should immediately be thinking pulmonary embolus (PE). A CT scan of the chest should be ordered urgently to confirm this suspicion, because this is a life-threatening emergency and treatment needs to be initiated rapidly.

Let us review the list of differential diagnoses of syncope that we identified in Chapter 5 to see how they relate to this patient's clinical presentation. This list is certainly not all inclusive, but it includes the most acute and most likely causes of syncope. Many diagnoses can usually be eliminated early in the evaluation of syncope. Often, however, the clinician is left with two or more possible diagnoses that can be confirmed or ruled out only through further evaluation.

**Differential Diagnoses of Syncope**

- Acute aortic dissection
- Aortic stenosis
- Bradyarrhythmias
- Brugada syndrome
- Cardiac tamponade
- Coronary artery disease/ischemia

- HCM
- Myocardial infarction
- Orthostatic syncope
- PAH
- PE
- Seizure/epilepsy

- Severe anemia
- Tachyarrhythmias
- TIA
- Vasovagal syncope

HCM, hypertrophic cardiomyopathy; PAH, pulmonary arterial hypertension; PE, pulmonary embolus; TIA, transient ischemic attack.

# PULLING IT ALL TOGETHER

## Working Through the Differential

As with the case scenario in Chapter 5, we can eliminate transient ischemic attack (TIA), seizure, and severe anemia right away in our patient based on the summary of information that follows. Although his syncopal event was not witnessed, it is unlikely he had a seizure because he had no evidence of tongue biting, incontinence, or symptoms of a postictal state.

- No neurological deficit
- No seizure-like activity (tongue biting, tonic–clonic movement, or incontinence)

- Rapid recovery to baseline
- Normal hemoglobin and hematocrit on CBC

Aortic dissection can also produce an elevated D-dimer level and syncope, as mentioned previously; however, another diagnosis is *more* likely, so we can move it down to the bottom of our list. We can eliminate cardiac tamponade altogether based on the following reasons:

- No widening of mediastinum
- Equal blood pressures in both arms
- No chest pain/back pain
- No jugular venous distention, pulsus paradoxus, or globular-shaped heart on chest film

This does *not* exclude the possibility that this patient may have a pericardial effusion. Rather, it simply indicates that he does not have signs consistent with cardiac tamponade from an effusion, and effusions in isolation do not tend to cause syncope unless there is hemodynamic compromise, as seen in cases of tamponade.

This patient has no clinical signs of an obstructive disease such as aortic stenosis. It is also unlikely that he has hypertrophic cardiomyopathy (HCM) based on clinical exam, but we cannot rule this out completely without an echocardiogram. These conditions are likely not the cause of his syncope based on the following:

- No murmur at rest and none noted with Valsalva
- No family history of cardiac disease or syncope
- Carotid upstrokes brisk, not delayed
- No prior history of syncope
- No ECG abnormalities suggestive of apical or left ventricular hypertrophy

Atrial fibrillation is a very common arrhythmia in HCM and even more so in patients with an outflow tract obstruction (Siontis et al., 2014). Some patients with HCM are also otherwise asymptomatic. This diagnosis is certainly a possibility in this patient, but less likely, so we can move it to the bottom of our list.

We learned in Chapter 5 that syncope and sudden cardiac death have been known to occur in patients with pulmonary hypertension (Mar et al., 2016). This patient is found to have an RV lift on exam and mild cardiomegaly, suggesting hypertrophy. If the clinical suspicion of PE is correct, this can cause RV dysfunction and subsequent pulmonary hypertension. So, while pulmonary hypertension may be present, it is likely a consequence of another issue, not the primary cause of his syncope.

What about vasovagal or orthostatic syncope? We have already learned that most episodes of syncope are either reflex mediated or due to orthostasis. This patient was hypotensive when EMS personnel arrived. His symptoms came on just after he stood and began clearing the table, suggesting some element of orthostasis. However, he was not orthostatic on evaluation in the emergency department.

If there is a PE, it can cause occlusion in the central pulmonary arteries and then partial resolution, causing transient hypotension and syncope (Altinsoy et al., 2016). This can make the diagnosis of PE difficult, because the blood pressure can normalize afterward. It is possible that the patient's syncopal spell was a result of a vasovagal event or orthostasis, but again this would likely be a consequence of the underlying issue and not the primary, isolated cause.

What about tachy- or bradyarrhythmias? We know the patient is tachycardic and in atrial fibrillation, but is this enough to cause syncope? Atrial fibrillation is unlikely to result in syncope, especially given that the patient's heart rate has not been extremely high. Certainly bradycardia or ventricular tachycardia can do so, but this patient has shown no signs of either. Myocardial infarction can precipitate ventricular arrhythmias but, again, aside from a positive troponin level, there are no other objective signs of ischemia. Atrial fibrillation is likely a manifestation of something else—in this case, the presence of a PE. Atrial fibrillation can occur as a consequence of PE by way of right atrial dilation from RV overload (Krajewska et al., 2017).

Brugada syndrome is characterized by the following:

- Coved ST-segment elevation in right precordial leads
- Incomplete right bundle branch block

There are no ECG findings in this patient consistent with this diagnosis; therefore, we can eliminate it as a possibility.

Syncope is unlikely to occur from myocardial ischemia in the absence of ECG changes as we learned in our previous scenario. There are features in this case that make myocardial infarction a possibility, such as:

- The presence of cardiovascular risk factors (obesity, hypertension, prior smoking history, borderline diabetes, and hyperlipidemia)
- A positive troponin level

However, this patient does not have any angina symptoms or ECG changes suggestive of ischemia. Although troponin levels are sensitive for myocardial injury, there are other causes for abnormal levels aside from this—which we have touched on in earlier chapters. Serial troponins must be checked to establish a typical rise and fall pattern that is seen with myocardial infarctions, or whether the levels remain flat. Since we have only one value at this time, we cannot completely rule out the presence of ischemia or infarction just yet. But, given the data, PE should be confirmed or excluded before a diagnosis of myocardial infarction is pursued.

So, let us talk about PE. The key objective feature that should have solidified this diagnosis at the top of the differential list is the positive D-dimer assay. The cardiovascular clinician already suspected PE during the evaluation, prompting the additional lab test to be ordered. Syncope can occur when there is sudden obstruction of the most proximal pulmonary arteries or a significant obstruction to cause reduction in cardiac output (Prandoni et al., 2016). Several other features and risk factors in this patient's presentation might have led you to think about PE as a possibility:

- Difficulty taking a deep breath and shortness of breath
- Presence of tachycardia (atrial fibrillation)
- Reduced oxygen saturation despite 4 L/min of oxygen in place
- Being overweight and possible sleep apnea
- Older age

Specific criteria that help determine the likelihood of a PE are summarized in the Wells criteria. It is widely used to quantify the risk of PE in patients in whom there is clinical suspicion of this diagnosis. Using this scoring system, as summarized by Boka (2016), we can determine the risk of PE based on this patient's presentation.

| Patient Findings | Clinical Probability of PE |
|---|---|
| Previous pulmonary embolus (PE) or deep vein thrombosis (DVT)-------------------------------------------+1.5 | *Low* = 0–1 |
| Heart rate >100 ------------------------------ +1.5 | *Intermediate* = 2–6 |
| Recent surgery or immobilization-------- +1.5 | *High* = ≥6 |
| Clinical signs of DVT-------------------------- +1.5 | |
| Alternative diagnosis less likely------------- +3 | |
| Hemoptysis-----------------------------------------+1 | |
| Cancer (treated within past 6 months)-----+1 | |

Based on the preceding scoring criteria, our patient has a score of 4.5. An alternative diagnosis is less likely given his elevated D-dimer value, along with the clinical presentation. If the D-dimer value was not available, the score would be only 1.5 for a heart rate of greater than 100. Often this scoring system is used only to determine risk in the absence of a D-dimer test. In the setting of a positive D-dimer result, imaging is typically pursued to confirm or rule out the presence of a PE regardless of the Wells score.

Another scoring system mentioned by Boka (2016) is the Geneva system, and its simplified (Revised Geneva) version. The Geneva system factors in age, limb pain, and heart rate ranges. It is comparable to the Wells criteria, but may be somwhat inferior according to some.

The classic symptoms of PE are chest pain, dypsnea, and hemoptysis (Altinsoy et al., 2016). Syncope is atypical as is abdominal pain and a new onset arrhythmia; however, it is important to remember that many patients do not present with classic signs of their conditions. We discussed earlier how syncope can occur in PE with transient hypotension. This patient certainly had transient hypotension surrounding his syncopal event.

Syncope in patients with acute PE is usually the result of acute right heart failure, hemodynamically unstable dysrhythmia, or vasovagal reflex, as mentioned by Altinsoy et al. (2016). Syncope in this setting is usually associated with a central or saddle PE, as well as elevated biomarkers and RV dysfunction. Often there are ECG abnormalities, such as an S wave in lead I, a Q wave in lead III, and a T wave in lead III (S1Q3T3) in the presence an acute PE, as well as T-wave inversions, but in as many instances, the ECG is completely normal with a submassive or massive PE. In our patient, the ECG demonstrated inverted T waves in the anterior leads (V1–V4). This finding, of course, could be a result of cardiac ischemia, but based on what we have learned it is further evidence to support a diagnosis of PE (Levis, 2011).

In addition, the risk of PE and atrial fibrillation increase with age. Atrial fibrillation may occur as a consequence of PE, as mentioned earlier, but it may also be a risk factor for PE (Krajewska et al., 2017) because lack of atrial contraction results in blood stasis and possible clot formation.

Troponin levels can be elevated in patients with PE. In an acute PE, cardiac troponins can be increased as a result of subendothelial ischemia in the right ventricle (Kilinc et al., 2012). Elevated troponin levels correlate with a greater degree of RV strain in submassive PEs compared with nonmassive PEs. Interestingly, dyspnea and syncope are more common with RV failure.

Let us summarize what we know to be true about this patient, and how the information supports a diagnosis of PE:

- New arrhythmia
- T-wave inversions in leads V1 to V4
- Elevated troponin, consistent with subendothelial ischemia in right ventricle
- Evidence of RV enlargement by exam and chest film (RV lift, cardiomegaly)
- Risk factors such as obesity and increased age
- Elevated D-dimer
- Hypoxia (an arterial blood gas reading would have helped to better quantify the degree of hypoxemia)

**Likely Diagnosis:** Acute PE

---

WHAT'S NEXT?

- Anticoagulation with unfractionated heparin is initiated.
- A stat CT scan of the chest is ordered, which confirms a submassive saddle PE.
- The patient is then given thrombolytic therapy, which results in improvement of symptoms.
- He is subsequently started on long-term anticoagulation.
- He converts back to normal sinus rhythm 48 hours after thrombolytic therapy is started.

---

# SUMMARIZING THE SCENARIO

In any patient who presents with a chief complaint of syncope, the history surrounding the event is imperative to determine the cause and ultimately the right treatment. We have emphasized this already. This patient did not present with what might be perceived as classic symptoms of a PE (i.e., chest pain, shortness of breath) or common antecedent risk factors (i.e., travel, surgery, cancer). The new arrhythmia as well as the positive troponin result led the first clinician to assume that atrial fibrillation or cardiac ischemia caused the event, when in fact it was a result of a larger, more acute issue.

The cardiovascular clinician focused on the details leading up to the event to determine whether the symptoms were abrupt in onset or had been ongoing, which we sometimes see with cardiac ischemia. In questioning the patient about his medical history, the consulting clinician was trying to determine risk for ischemia as a culprit. Knowing that this patient remained in distress despite a modestly elevated heart rate should have raised suspicion that the rhythm abnormality was not the primary issue. This is what prompted the addition of a D-dimer lab test. Although the D-dimer can be elevated in other conditions, the clinical picture was most consistent with a PE. This ultimately led to prompt imaging to confirm the diagnosis and may have saved the patient's life.

Clinicians often get caught up in the objective evidence and overlook the clinical picture. If a diagnosis of cardiac ischemia had been pursued, this patient would likely have received unfractionated heparin based on protocol, and serial troponins as well as ECGs would have been obtained to further assess his condition. The troponin levels likely would have remained flat, prompting an alternative diagnosis to be pursued. It is reasonable to assume, given the size of the PE, that anticoagulation alone would not have been sufficient to treat it and his condition might have deteriorated before an accurate diagnosis was made.

As experts in the field, cardiovascular clinicians must think outside the box and consider all possible diagnoses even when the presentation does not fit the classic mold. A D-dimer test and imaging should be obtained for any patient who presents with a new arrhythmia, low oxygenation, and syncope to evaluate for the possibility of a PE. A submassive PE can cause more atypical symptoms than a nonmassive PE and can lead to abrupt hemodynamic compromise and death if not treated promptly.

## COMMON PITFALLS AND ASSUMPTIONS

Syncope is one of those vague chief complaints that can result from a wide variety of underlying problems. Often, patients define syncope as a "near faint" without actual loss of consciousness. As clinicians, we must always first determine whether or not there was actual loss of consciousness and not a perception of such. In addition, questioning witnesses is key to helping to determine whether any seizure-like activity or neurological deficit was associated with the event. This information can lead to a completely different workup.

Loss of consciousness related to a neurological event is different than frank syncope, as we have learned in this chapter. Asking patients about symptoms leading up to the event and their mental state after resuming consciousness can be one of the most important pieces of information gathered during the evaluation.

Syncope can be the result of a fairly benign condition, or one that is life threatening; the devil is in the details. In the case scenario in Chapter 5, it would have been easy to dismiss the patient's episode of syncope as dehydration or bradycardia in a seemingly fit woman. A thorough clinical exam and a deeper understanding into her history resulted in a much more complex cause to her syncope. In this scenario, the same is true. It may have been easy to dismiss the patient's episode of syncope as transient hypotension related to his atrial fibrillation. However, he remained unwell despite improvement in blood pressure, and other objective evidence supported the conclusion that there was more to the story than the initial presentation suggested.

It is of utmost importance that clinicians focus on the whole picture and not be derailed by a few abnormal lab values. Emergency department providers do not have the expertise of cardiovascular specialists; their job is to promptly identify what is occurring and treat patients accordingly. Often the presence of an abnormal rhythm or lab value can narrow the provider's focus, leading to misdiagnosis, rather than being viewed as one piece as evidence that is part of a larger whole.

In addition, the utilization of scoring systems can be misleading. If a Wells score had been calculated for this patient before obtaining the D-dimer result, he would have fallen into the low-risk category, again highlighting the importance of considering the clinical context. When cardiovascular clinicians are called upon to assist in complex cases, it is imperative that we recognize this and conduct the history and exam based on this concept. Each piece of evidence should prompt additional questioning or testing to exclude and ultimately confirm the right diagnosis.

# REFERENCES

Altinsoy, B., Erboy, F., Tanriverdi, H., Uygur, F., Ornek, T., Atalay, F., ... Tor, M. (2016) Syncope as a presentation of acute pulmonary embolism. *Therapeutics and Clinical Risk Management, 12*, 1023–1028.

Boka, K., (2016). Pumonary embolism clinical scoring systems. Retrieved from : http://emedicine.medscape.com/srticle/1918940-overview.

Kilinc, G., Dogan, O., Berk, S., Epozturk, Ozsahin, S., Akkurt, I., (2012). Significance of serum cardiac troponin I levels in pulmonary emoblism. Journal of Thoracic Disease, 4(6), 588-593.

Krajewska, A., Ptaszynska-Kopczynska, K., Kiluk, I., Kosacka, U., Milewski, R., Krajewski, J., ... Sobkowicz, B. (2017). Paroxysmal atrial fibrillation in the course of acute pulmonary embolism: Clinical significance and impact on prognosis. *Biomedical Research International, 2017.*5049802 doi:10.1155/2017/5049802

Levis, J. (2011). ECG diagnosis: Pulmonary embolism. *The Permanente Journal, 15*(4), 75.

Mar, P., Nwazue, V., Black, B., Biaggioni, I., Diedrich, A., Oaranjape, S., ...Hemnes, A., (2016). Valsalva Maneuver in Pulmonary Arterial Hypertension: Susceptibility to Syncope and Autonomic Dysfuncion. *Chest*, 149(5), 1252–1260. http://dx.doi.org/10.1016/j.chest.2015.11.015.

Parwani, A., Boldt, L., Huemer, M., Wutzler, A., Blaschke, D., Rolf, S., ... Haverkamp, W. (2013). Atrial fibrillation-induced cardiac troponin I release. *International Journal of Cardiology*, 168(3), 2734–2737. doi:10.1016/j.icard.2013.03.087

Patel, P., & Quinn, J. (2015). Syncope: A review of emergency department management and disposition. *Clinical and Experimental Emergency Medicine*, 2(2), 67–74.

Pathak, V., Rendon, I., & Muthyala, P. (2011). Elevated D-dimer is not always pulmonary embolism. *Respiratory Medicine CME*, 4(2), 91–92. doi:10.1016/j.rmedc.2010.05.006

Prandoni, P., Anthonie, W., Lensing, M., Prins, M., Ciammaichella, M., Perlati, M., ... Barbar, S. (2016). Prevalence of pulmonary emoblism among patients hospitalized for syncope. *New England Journal of Medicine*, 375, 1524–1531. doi:10.1056/NEJMoa162172

Siontis, K., Geske, J., Ong, K., Nishimura, R., Ommen, S., Gersh, B. (2014). Atrial fibrillation in hypertrophic cardiomyopathy: Prevalence, clinical correlations, and mortality in a large high-risk population. *Journal of the American Heart Association*, 3(3). doi:10.1161.JHAH.114.001002

# CHAPTER 7

# Elevated Troponin: A First Look

## DEFINITION AND SIGNIFICANCE OF TROPONINS

According to *Farlex Medical Dictionary* (2012), troponin is a "globular protein of muscle that binds to tropomyosin and is a central regulatory protein of muscle contraction." Three components make up the troponin complex: troponin I (TnI), troponin T (TnT), and troponin C (TnC).

Troponin I and troponin T are found in cardiac and skeletal muscles. They are encoded by different genes in both types of muscles, creating the distinction between the two types of proteins (Ru, Xiao, Ye, & Ping 2013). Specific assays are available for both troponin I and troponin T, but because troponin C and skeletal troponin C are identical, no assays have been developed for this component. Both troponin I and troponin T are used to diagnose heart attacks. The primary difference between the two is that troponin I measures only cardiac troponin whereas troponin T may cross-react with troponin found in other muscles and give false positive results in the absence of heart damage (troponins test; Mosby's Medical Dictionary, 2009).

Troponins have long since been the preferred biomarker of choice in detecting cardiac injury as seen in myocardial infarctions (MIs). Most clinical investigators believe the release of troponin is a specific indicator of myocardial damage. Current modern assays detect myocardial damage with a resultant rise in troponin levels within 3 to 4 hours after injury (Mangla & Gupta 2015).

Cardiac troponins have a sensitivity higher than 95% and a specificity of 90% for detecting myocardial injury (Sabatine & Cannon, 2015), making false positive elevations rare. The European Society of Cardiology (ESC) along with the American College of Cardiology (ACC) developed a universal definition of an acute MI in 2012 as defined as follows (Thygesen et al., 2012):

1. Detection of a rise and fall of cardiac biomarkers along with *one* of the following:

   a. Symptoms

   b. Pathological Q waves on ECG

   c. New or presumed new ST–T-wave changes or new left bundle branch block (LBBB)

   d. Identification of a coronary thrombus by autopsy or angiogram

   e. Imaging evidence of new loss of myocardium or regional wall motion abnormalities

This is the primary definition; however, there are other situations in which an acute MI can also be diagnosed, such as cardiac death with symptoms suggestive of ischemia prior to biomarkers being obtained, percutaneous coronary intervention (PCI)–related MI, coronary artery bypass grafting (CABG)–related MI, and stent thrombosis–associated MI (Thygesen et al., 2012).

The ESC and the ACC joint task force went on to further define MI based on the mechanism by which it occurs to help in distinguishing classic MI from other causes of troponin elevation. Four types of MI were identified, but most cases fall into either type I or type II. These are defined as follows:

- *Type I*: A spontaneous MI consequent to a pathological process in the coronary artery wall, such as plaque rupture, erosion, or dissection

- *Type II*: An MI secondary to an ischemic imbalance due to high oxygen demand or decreased supply such as coronary spasm, coronary embolus, anemia, and alterations in heart rate or blood pressure

It is often quite difficult to distinguish between type I and type II MI. Type II MI is more often a diagnosis of exclusion. As we have seen in earlier chapters, troponin levels can be elevated in conditions other than MI, such as myopericarditis, pulmonary embolus, and renal disease, to name a few. In such cases, the presence of an elevated troponin level is more useful for prognosis than diagnosis. Collinson and Lindahl (2016) identify the following key features that help in diagnosing a type II MI:

- Features inconsistent with type I

- Increased and changing troponin value

- Presence of a clinical condition known to increase oxygen demand or decrease supply

- Confounding clinical condition or comorbidities that are potentially associated or known to be associated with myocardial injury

- The absence of symptoms or signs indicating other nonischemic causes of troponin elevations (e.g., myocarditis)

Recently, high-sensitivity troponin assays have become available that enable detection at lower concentrations, improving diagnostic accuracy for ruling in or out an acute MI. These have been used in Asia and Europe and were approved in the United States at the beginning of 2017. The high-sensitivity assays obviate the need for serial testing every 3 hours (as is current practice), enabling a zero to 1-hour approach (Westermann, Neuman, Sörensen, & Blankenberg, 2017). The current ESC guidelines recommend this approach for early discrimination of an acute MI, as these assays have excellent negative predictive values for events at 1 hour (Roffi et al., 2015). MIs can thus be ruled in or out with a single blood draw rather than serial measurements.

The use of high-sensitivity troponins will certainly allow for earlier identification of an acute MI, but they will also increase identification of type II MI as well as other conditions in which troponin elevation can be present. This can lead to potentially more testing and greater cost to this group of patients.

In previous chapters, we discussed common chief complaints for which cardiovascular clinicians are often consulted. Elevated troponin levels are not a chief complaint, but rather an objective finding that represent one of the most common reasons cardiologists and cardiovascular practitioners are consulted in an acute care setting. We are often asked to interpret the meaning of these values and determine whether or not these values represent the presence of a classic MI, type II MI, or another cause altogether.

The history and clinical context remain crucial in helping to identify the cause of the troponin rise; however, in most cases it is primarily the serial trend of the troponin levels, EKGs, and imaging that lead to a diagnosis.

Since earlier chapters have already presented scenarios in which the troponin level can be abnormal in the presence or absence of an MI, this chapter and Chapter 8 are designed somewhat differently. Additional cases are presented and discussed but two provider histories are not compared because the involvement of the cardiovascular clinician is not due to a subjective complaint with clinical suspicion of a diagnosis, but rather due to an objective finding with a diagnosis that is already being pursued.

## CASE SCENARIO

Cardiology is called at 1 p.m. for a STEMI alert in a 62-year-old White female who presented to the emergency department with complaints of substernal chest pain and pressure that started around 11 a.m. She reports profound emotional distress as a result of her husband's death 2 days ago in a car accident. She awoke this morning with vague nausea and noticed the chest pressure beginning around 11 a.m. as she was discussing funeral arrangements with her family. She thought it was anxiety, but the pain persisted without relief so her family brought her to the emergency department for further evaluation and treatment.

She has no history of coronary artery disease but does have a past medical history of hypertension, for which she takes lisinopril, 10 mg daily. Her mother had ovarian cancer and died in her 60s. Her father is in his 80s with hypertension, hyperlipidemia, and kidney disease. She is a lifelong nonsmoker. She drinks an occasional glass of wine with dinner. She does not use any illicit drugs.

On arrival to the emergency department her blood pressure was 143/74 mmHg in the right arm, 146/80 mmHg in the left arm, pulse was

*(continued)*

## CASE SCENARIO (continued)

78 beats per minute, respiratory rate was 16 breaths per minute, and oxygen saturation was 97% on room air. She was afebrile. An ECG was obtained and showed ST-segment elevation in anterior leads, V3 through V5. A basic chemistry panel, CBC, and troponin level were ordered. The STEMI alert was made after completion of the ECG. A chest film was performed and did not show any acute findings. The exam was unremarkable for any clinical signs of heart failure or other abnormalities. The patient was hemodynamically stable.

It is confirmed that the patient has no history of bleeding disorders or active bleeding issues. She is not taking any blood thinners or anti-platelet agents. She is subsequently given guideline-directed therapy with heparin; ticagrelor, 180 mg; chewable aspirin, 324 mg; and nitro-glycerin sublingual.

She is taken to the catheterization lab urgently for coronary angiogra-phy. The troponin I level comes back at 0.39 ng/mL. Coronary angiography shows no obstructive coronary artery disease. A left ventriculogram shows apical ballooning. An echocardiogram demonstrates an EF of 35% with api-cal akinesis consistent with stress-induced, or Takotsubo, cardiomyopathy.

The patient is admitted, and her troponin levels trend to 0.47 ng/mL, then peak at 0.50 ng/mL. Her pain subsides without recur-rence, and the ECG transitions over the next few days from ST elevation to diffuse T-wave abnormalities. She is started on appro-priate medical therapy with a beta-blocker, aspirin, and statin; con-tinued on her previously prescribed lisinopril; and discharged 3 days after admission. A follow-up echocardiogram 3 weeks later shows complete resolution of her cardiomyopathy.

CBC, complete blood count; EF, ejection fraction; STEMI, ST-segment elevation myocardial infarction.

## KEY FEATURES OF THE HISTORY

When a patient has evidence of ST elevation (localized to specific leads and not global) on ECG and associated chest pain, the diagnosis is an acute ST-segment elevation myocardial infarction (STEMI) until proven otherwise. Obtaining the history can help support this diagnosis but does not change the initial management in these cases. Eliciting a detailed history in this setting can be difficult because the provider may not have much time with the patient before he or she is whisked to coronary angiography. It is important to get the most information possible during this time.

The most important information to identify is whether the patient has known coronary artery disease, what the risk factors are, and what events took place surrounding the symptom onset. It is also important to assess whether the patient is on blood thinning medication or antiplatelet medication, whether he or she had bleeding issues, and whether any upcoming surgeries or procedures are planned. These important details are factored in if the patient requires a stent during coronary angiography. This information will help determine whether patients can safely receive a coronary intervention with a stent if necessary, whether they can take required medication afterward, and what kind of stent can be used.

This patient arrived at the emergency department with complaints of chest pain and nausea that preceded the pain. She had no history of coronary artery disease and had been experiencing the pain for a couple of hours prior to presentation. In this case scenario one of the most important details is the mention of an extremely stressful event—the recent death of her husband. This should prompt the clinician to consider whether the patient has stress-induced cardiomyopathy, also known as Takotsubo cardiomyopathy. This is a diagnosis of exclusion, however, and STEMI must be ruled out first.

## KEY FEATURES OF THE DATA

The initial key objective data in this case scenario are the ECG and, to a lesser extent, the troponin value. The ST-segment elevation prompted the call to cardiology. The presence of an elevated troponin level further supported the suspicion that this was likely STEMI. As cardiology providers, however, we know that Takotsubo cardiomyopathy presents identically to STEMI but has distinct features on echocardiogram and left ventriculogram.

As more information was obtained, the coronary angiography results became the most relevant data, completely eliminating STEMI as a diagnosis. The stressful event, along with the apical ballooning found on echocardiogram and left ventriculogram, supported the diagnosis of Takotsubo cardiomyopathy.

## DIFFERENTIALS AND DIFFERENCES IN EXAM

In the setting of a suspected STEMI, often the exam is focused on identifying whether there is any hemodynamic instability and any signs of arrhythmia, heart failure, or adventitious lung or heart sounds. This patient's vital signs were stable without any major discrepancy in each arm and there were no abnormal exam findings. Her heart rhythm was sinus and she was oxygenating adequately on room air.

Despite the critical and often time-sensitive presentation of STEMI, it is important that other acute issues be identified before the patient undergoes coronary angiography. This process typically takes place simultaneously while the interventional team is being notified and the patient is being prepared to go to the catheterization lab. In this scenario, blood pressures were taken in each arm to ensure no aortic dissection was present and chest film confirmed no abnormalities, such as a widened mediastinum, heart failure, or any other significant findings. These findings help to support the course of action and better quantify the risk for the procedure if any other abnormalities were found.

Many conditions can cause elevated troponin levels in the absence of acute coronary syndromes. We have discussed some of these in previous chapters. Let us look further at some of the differential diagnoses for elevated troponin levels according to Januzzi (2010).

## PULLING IT ALL TOGETHER

### Working Through the Differential

In earlier chapters, we discussed how troponin elevation can be present in renal disease, myopericarditis, and pulmonary embolus. In the case scenario for this chapter, the cause of the troponin elevation was identified quickly owing to the nature of the presentation. Diagnosis is not always

Differential Diagnoses of Elevated Troponin Levels

| | | |
|---|---|---|
| • Acute MI | • Embolus | • Myocarditis or pericarditis |
| • Acute stroke | • Endocarditis | • Pulmonary |
| • Amyloidosis | • Endurance exercise | • Renal disease |
| • Anemia | • Gastrointestinal bleeding | • Rhabdomyolysis |
| • Aortic dissection | • Head trauma | • Scleroderma |
| • Arrhythmia | • Heart failure | • Sepsis |
| • Cardiac procedures | • Hemochromatosis | • Takotsubo cardiomyopathy |
| • Drug reaction | • Hypertension or hypotension | |

MI, myocardial infarction.

this clear-cut, however, and it is important to consider possibilities other than an MI if the clinical picture does not support it.

This case is a nice example of troponin elevation in the absence of either a true type I or type II MI. Takotsubo cardiomyopathy is found in 1% to 2% of troponin-positive patients who are suspected of having an acute coronary syndrome (Falk & Hersberger, 2015). It is thought to be due to a catecholamine surge that results in microvascular dysfunction and inflammatory activation (Horowitz & Nguyen, 2014).

Takotsubo cardiomyopathy is more common in women, and there is usually an antecedent emotional trigger leading to the presentation. It should always be part of the differential diagnosis when women present with an acute coronary syndrome. Takotsubo cardiomyopathy can mimic a STEMI presentation, as seen in this scenario. Typically, there is troponin elevation, but to a lesser degree than would be seen with a true STEMI. Studies have looked at ECG abnormalities in Takotsubo cardiomyopathy and STEMI in an attempt to differentiate the two, but ultimately the ECG alone cannot confirm the presence of Takotsubo cardiomyopathy and, owing to the negative impact of prolonging coronary angiography in the presence of ST elevation, it remains the test of choice to confirm the diagnosis. Other studies have looked at the presence of circulating catecholamines in STEMI patients and patients with Takotsubo cardiomyopathy, and nearly 75% of patients with the latter had elevations higher than those seen in patients with STEMI (Tomich, 2017).

The Mayo Clinic developed criteria for the diagnosis of Takotsubo cardiomyopathy in 2004, and revised them in 2008. The presence of all four of the following criteria must be met (Prasad, Lerman, & Rihal, 2008):

1. Transient hypokinesis, akinesis, or dyskinesis of the left ventricular mid-segments with or without apical involvement; the regional wall motion abnormalities extend beyond a single epicardial vascular distribution; a stressful trigger is often but not always present

2. Absence of obstructive coronary artery disease or angiographic evidence of acute plaque rupture

3. New ECG abnormalities (ST-segment elevation or T-wave inversion), or modest elevation in cardiac troponin

4. Absence of pheochromocytoma and myocarditis

Takotsubo cardiomyopathy is a temporary condition that results in normalization of EF within days to weeks.

**Likely Diagnosis:** Takotsubo cardiomyopathy

---

WHAT'S NEXT?

- The resolution of this case was described earlier. At the time of the patient's 3-week follow-up appointment, her cardiac function had normalized.

---

# SUMMARIZING THE SCENARIO

This case scenario seemed to be a classic presentation of STEMI based on the ECG findings and the patient's symptoms. Prompt evaluation and coronary angiography proved that she in fact did not have an MI, but rather Takotsubo cardiomyopathy precipitated by profound emotional stress. The history should have led you to consider this as a possibility even though STEMI had to be ruled out.

Most STEMI presentations do not have elevated troponin levels at the time they are drawn initially in the emergency department. As discussed in earlier chapters, the current assays used do not detect myocardial injury for 3 to 4 hours. In classic presentations of acute coronary syndromes, patients develop chest pain or discomfort worrisome enough for them to seek medical attention not long after onset. The initial troponin level typically is obtained within that 3- to 4-hour time frame of onset of pain, leading to undetectable levels on the first blood draw. In our case scenario, the patient had symptoms for 2 hours before presentation, and the initial troponin level was already elevated. This agrees with information reported by Tomich (2017), who noted that troponin levels were elevated in 90% of patients with Takotsubo cardiomyopathy and, in addition, elevated at the time of admission.

Researchers have attempted to identify patterns present on ECG, ratios of various biomarkers, and other features of Takotsubo cardiomyopathy to try to differentiate it from an acute coronary syndrome; however, coronary angiography remains the gold standard to firmly diagnose the condition. Coronary artery disease may be present in patients who manifest Takotsubo cardiomyopathy; however, it is the absence of *obstructive* disease and the presence of myocardial inflammation that ultimately confirms this diagnosis.

If this patient had presented without evidence of STEMI, the clinical suspicion of Takotsubo cardiomyopathy could have been further supported by an early imaging study such as an echocardiogram. This would have demonstrated apical akinesis consistent with a picture of apical ballooning syndrome, or Takotsubo cardiomyopathy. Although coronary angiography would still have been necessary to eliminate the possibility that ischemic heart disease had a role in the patient's symptoms, MI would have become second on the differential list to Takotsubo cardiomyopathy, rather than the primary working diagnosis, which in turn would have changed the prognostic implications.

Takotsubo cardiomyopathy has become more widely understood since it was first reported. It should be considered in any patient presenting with symptoms consistent with acute coronary syndrome and a precipitating stressful event. Keep in mind the stressful event does not need to be negative and does not always have to be an emotional trigger. Physical stressors such as an acute illness with associated cardiac symptoms should also raise the suspicion that Takotsubo cardiomyopathy is a possible cause.

In Chapter 8, we review another case involving elevated troponin levels that leads to a more extensive workup, and a much different diagnosis.

## REFERENCES

Collinson, P., & Lindahl, B. (2016). Diagnosing type 2 myocardial infarction. *American College of Cardiology Expert Analysis*.

Falk, R., & Hersberger, R. (2015). The dilated, restrictive, and infiltrative cardiomyopathies. In *Braunwald's heart disease: A textbook of cardiovascular medicine* (10th ed.). Philadelphia, PA: Elsevier/Saunders.

Farlex Partner Medical Dictionary. (2012). Troponin. Retrieved from http://medical-dictionary.thefreedictionary.com/troponin

Horowitz, J., & Nguyen, T. (2014). Differentiating Tako-Tsubo cardiomyopathy from myocardial infarction. *ESC Council for Cardiology Practice, 13*(7).

Januzzi Jr., J. (2010). Causes of non-ACS related troponin elevations. *American College of Cardiology*. Retrieved from http://www.acc.org/latest-in-cardiology/articles/2014/07/18/13/16/causes-of-non-acs-related-troponin-elevations

Mangla, A., & Gupta, A. (2015). Troponins. Retrieved from http://emedicine.medscape.com/article/2073935-overview

Mosby's Medical Dictionary, 8th edition. (2009). Troponins test. Retrieved from http://medical-dictionary.thefreedictionary.com/troponins+test

Prasad, A., Lerman, A., & Rihal, C. (2008). Apical ballooning syndrome (TakoTsubo or stress cardiomyopathy): A mimic of acute myocardial infarction. *American Heart Journal, 155*, 408–417.

Roffi, M., Patrono, C., Collet, J., Mueller, C., Valgimigli, M., Andreotti, F., ... Luis Zamorano, J. (2015). European Society of Cariology (ESC) guidelines for the management of acute coronary syndromes in patients presenting without persistent ST-segment elevation. Task Force for the Management of Acute Coronary Syndromes in patients presenting without persistent ST segment elevation of the ESC. *European Heart Journal, 37*, 267–315.

Ru, Y., Xioa, F., Ye, Y., & Ping, Y. (2013). High sensitivity cardiac troponin T. *Journal of Geriatric Cardiology, 10*(1), 102–109.

Sabatine, M., Cannon, C. (2015). Approach to the Patient with Chest Pain .In D. L. Mann, D. P. Sipes, P. Libby, & R. O. Bonow, *Braunwald's Heart Disease: A textbook of Cardiovascular Medicine* (10th ed., pp. 1057–1067). Philadelphia, PA: Elsevier/Saunders.

Thygesen, K., Alpert, J., Jaffe, A., Simoons, M., Chitman, B., & White, H. (2012). Third universal definition of myocardial infarction. *Circulation, 126*(16), 2020–2035.

Tomich, E. (2017). Takotsubo cariomyopathy workup. Retrieved from http://emedicine.medscape.com/article/1513631-workup#c7

Westermann, D., Neumann, T., Sörensen, N., & Blankenberg, S. (2017). High-sensitivity assays for troponin in patients with cardiac disease. *Nature Reviews Cardiology, 14*, 472–483. doi:10.1038/nrcardio.2017.48

# CHAPTER 8

# Elevated Troponin: Another Encounter

In this chapter, as in Chapter 7, we examine a patient scenario involving elevated troponin levels and explore various causes for the patient's presentation. Elevated troponin is not a symptom but rather an objective finding that triggers input and evaluation by cardiovascular clinicians on a regular basis.

## CASE SCENARIO

A 41-year-old White male presents to the emergency department with complaints of fevers, lethargy, and nighttime sweating. He also reports shortness of breath with exertion, and weight loss of 20 lb over the past 3 months. He initially experienced these symptoms 6 months ago and began going to the gym and working out, thinking his symptoms were due to deconditioning; however, the exertional dyspnea ultimately led him to stop these activities.

Over the past 2 months his symptoms have progressed. He has lost a total of 60 lb over the course of a year. He has had difficulty carrying out activities of daily living without becoming profoundly short of breath. He has experienced falls from weakness as well as confusion at times. His symptoms

*(continued)*

## CASE SCENARIO *(continued)*

have resulted in frequent absences from work. He was evaluated recently at another hospital and is unclear about the details, but reports that he was diagnosed with anemia and associated tachycardia and placed on a beta-blocker.

He is brought into the emergency department by a friend who went to check on him and found him appearing to be very ill, with some alterations in speech that prompted the friend to bring him for evaluation. He has no significant past medical history or other family history. He drinks socially, amounting to two or three beers per week. He does not use illicit drugs. He smoked tobacco for about 10 years and quit 9 years ago. His only medication is atenolol, 25 mg daily.

On presentation to the emergency department, he is febrile with a temperature of 38.1°C, his pulse is 117 beats per minute, blood pressure is 94/45 mmHg, respiratory rate is 22 breaths per minute, and oxygen saturation is 100% on room air. An ECG is obtained that shows sinus tachycardia with non-specific ST–T-wave abnormalities. His initial laboratory values are remarkable for hemoglobin of 7.8 mg/dL, hematocrit of 24.2%, white blood cell count of 13,600, and platelet count of 77,000. His sedimentation rate is elevated at 47 mm/hr, and his blood chemistry is notable only for a creatinine level of 1.3 mg/dL. Liver function studies show ALT of 149 U/L, AST of 217 U/L, and ALP of 119 U/L. His exam is notable for a grade IV/VI diastolic murmur, decreased peripheral perfusion, and ataxia. A chest film demonstrates small pleural effusions but no infectious or inflammatory process.

The patient is admitted to the medicine service for concerns of hematological malignancy with sepsis. Broad-spectrum antibiotics are initiated. Initial testing includes blood cultures and viral studies, as well as imaging with echocardiogram and CT scans of the head, chest, abdomen, and pelvis.

Within 12 hours the patient becomes more anemic, with rising fevers and persistent hypotension. An ECG is obtained that demonstrates delayed

*(continued)*

## CASE SCENARIO

R-wave progression, worsening ST–T-wave abnormalities in the inferolateral leads, and some ST depression laterally. This prompts an order for the troponin T level to be drawn; it is elevated at 0.48 ng/mL. A cardiology consult is arranged at that point.

The exam performed by the consulting cardiologist is notable for murmur consistent with aortic regurgitation, as noted earlier. The patient is questioned about any dental procedures or other invasive procedures within the last year and denies having such. No splinter hemorrhages, petechiae, Janeway lesions, or Osler's nodes are present.

Serial troponin levels are 0.45 ng/mL and 0.49 ng/mL, respectively. Blood cultures are positive for *Streptococcus viridians*. Imaging of the head reveals subacute parietal infarcts, and CT scan of the abdomen shows a splenic infarct. Echocardiogram demonstrates a preserved ejection fraction of 54% and a bicuspid aortic valve, with severe regurgitation and flow reversal into the abdominal and thoracic aorta. A dense mobile vegetation is present on the aortic valve consistent with infective endocarditis. A transesophageal echocardiogram (TEE) is obtained; it confirms a large mobile vegetation of the aortic valve with perivalvular abscess.

The patient is then transported for emergent aortic valve replacement. He continues to be anemic postoperatively, with evidence of a large gastrointestinal bleed, and subsequently undergoes upper endoscopy. This procedure identifies a duodenal ulcer that is then treated. He does well afterward and recovery is uneventful. He is ultimately discharged home after a nearly 3-week stay.

## KEY FEATURES OF THE HISTORY

The patient is a fairly young man who presented with months of fever, night sweats, weight loss, anemia, and shortness of breath. These symptoms were quite concerning for an underlying malignancy that was initially suspected. These are also common symptoms in patients with endocarditis; however, nothing in his history suggested a primary cardiac issue, which is why cardiac enzymes were not initially obtained. The mild abnormalities seen on ECG at the time of admission were also not worrisome enough to suspect ischemia as the culprit.

Endocarditis can result any time bacteria enter the bloodstream; most commonly this is a result of a dental procedure, intravenous drug use, or an invasive procedure. Typically, the body is able to fight off the bacteria; however, certain underlying heart conditions, such as congenital abnormalities, artificial valves, or mechanical devices can predispose individuals to developing endocarditis.

Once a murmur was identified the patient was asked whether he had undergone any procedures or performed any activities that might have increased his risk for infection. He had not. So, although often there is some relationship between the two, it is not always the case.

Anytime a patient presents with symptoms such as these, endocarditis should be considered in the differential. Appropriate testing and imaging was ordered to thoroughly evaluate the patient and identify a source of his symptoms. The key features in his history that prompted troponin levels to be drawn were the rapid decline in his condition and the changes noted on ECG.

This patient had multiple symptoms that could be representative of a number of problems, so it was not unreasonable to evaluate further for possible ischemia. However, in this case, the cause of the abnormal troponin levels was likely multifactorial. We discuss this further in the next section.

# KEY FEATURES OF THE DATA

The most important pieces of data in a patient who is suspected of having endocarditis are the echocardiogram and the transesophageal echocardiogram (TEE). This patient presented with multiple symptoms and signs of infection; therefore, imaging of the brain, chest, and abdomen were ordered appropriately. Subacute infarcts were present in the brain, and splenic infarcts were also noted, which should raise suspicion of a cardioembolic source as the causative mechanism. Echocardiogram confirmed the presence of a vegetation on the aortic valve, which was then better visualized by TEE.

The troponin level and ECG are not key features of the data in this case scenario. The abnormal troponin levels play more of a prognostic role, but do not alter or change the course of treatment. The pattern of troponin levels in this patient was not the typical rise and fall pattern seen with myocardial injury. In a different clinical context, further testing to establish the presence of significant coronary artery disease might have been pursued; however, this patient was hemodynamically unstable and needed emergent surgical intervention.

This patient also had ongoing anemia, which is noteworthy. It has been well established that valvular disease such as aortic stenosis with associated gastrointestinal bleeding can be a result of acquired von Willebrand syndrome (AVWS) in such patients (Wan, Liang, Vaidya, Blackshear, & Chen, 2014). Rare case reports have noted the same for mitral and aortic regurgitation. This patient was evaluated for AVWS and the result was negative. Ultimately his anemia was corrected once the bleeding ulcer was identified and treated.

His blood cultures came back positive for viridians group *Streptococcus*, which is the most common cause of native valve endocarditis (Baddour, Freeman, Rakesh, Wilson, & Wilson, 2015). In addition, he was found to have a bicuspid aortic valve, which was likely the preexisting congenital abnormality that put him at increased risk of developing infective endocarditis. According to Baddour and colleagues (2015), regurgitant lesions are more prone to infection than stenotic ones, and aortic valve regurgitation is the lesion second only to mitral valve prolapse that is predisposed to developing endocarditis.

# DIFFERENTIALS AND DIFFERENCES IN EXAM

The key feature in this patient's exam was the presence of a significant murmur. This led to the suspicion that infective endocarditis could be the source of his protracted symptoms. Once this condition was suspected, the cardiovascular clinician evaluated the patient for signs of systemic embolization looking for splinter hemorrhages, Osler's nodes, and Janeway lesions—none of which were found.

Differential Diagnoses of Elevated Troponin Levels

- Acute MI
- Acute stroke
- Amyloidosis
- Anemia
- Aortic dissection
- Arrhythmia
- Cardiac procedures
- Drug reaction

- Endocarditis
- Endurance exercise
- Gastrointestinal bleeding
- Head trauma
- Heart failure
- Hemochromatosis
- Hypertension or hypotension
- Myocarditis or pericarditis

- Pulmonary embolus
- Rhabdomyolysis
- Renal disease
- Scleroderma
- Sepsis
- Takotsubo cardiomyopathy

MI, myocardial infarction.

The presence of a murmur with associated fevers, nighttime sweating, and weight loss should raise the clinical suspicion of endocarditis to the top of your differential list. The troponin levels were drawn on this patient because of more profound ECG changes in the setting of hemodynamic compromise—providing another example of how ischemia is not always a cause for elevated troponins.

Let us review the differential diagnosis list for troponin elevation that we previously studied in Chapter 7 (Januzzi, 2010).

# PULLING IT ALL TOGETHER

## Working Through the Differential

Troponin levels can be elevated in the presence of sepsis, gastrointestinal bleeding, and endocarditis—all of which were noted in this patient. Do you think that one of these was more likely to have caused the elevated troponin levels than the others, or did the elevation likely result from a combination of the three?

Higher levels of troponin in patients with infective endocarditis have been studied and indicate a less favorable prognosis. Some researchers suggest that myocardial damage can occur in this setting due to local invasion and abscess formation at the primary site of infection (Thoker, Khan, Rashid, & Zafar, 2016). Thoker and colleagues also suggest that coronary embolization can occur or subclinical septic microemboli can enter the coronary artery anatomy, causing microinfarcts. The mechanism has yet to be clearly defined.

Troponin elevation is common among septic patients, but the cause is not well understood. Potential causes of myocardial dysfunction in septic patients include demand ischemia, cardiac myotoxic effects, or reactive oxygen radicals and alterations in coronary blood flow (Sheyin, Davies, Duan, & Perez, 2015). Sepsis is typically not a consequence of coronary obstruction from underlying atherosclerosis. It was found in patients who died a septic-related death that while all had increased postmortem troponin levels, none had coronary artery disease, heart failure, or myocardial damage (Tettamanti, Hervet, Grabherr, & Palmiere, 2016).

Elevated troponin levels can be found in the presence of a (gastrointestinal) bleed as a result of demand ischemia. In the presence of anemia, there is decreased oxygen-carrying capacity, hypovolemia, hypotension, and tachycardia, all of which can cause some myocardial ischemia. This can be classified as a type II myocardial infarction (MI). This patient presented with all of these features but did not have a straightforward gastrointestinal bleed. The presence of sepsis and infective endocarditis contributed to the elevated troponin levels.

The identification and diagnosis of endocarditis occurred fairly quickly from the time of presentation to the time of treatment. Infective endocarditis can be deadly, and it is imperative to initiate treatment and continue the evaluation based on clinical suspicion alone in order to avoid hemodynamic compromise.

The definitive diagnosis of infective endocarditis is determined by positive blood cultures and the presence of an abscess or intracardiac vegetation. The Duke criteria have been used for many years to establish a diagnosis of endocarditis. To make the diagnosis the following findings must be present: Two major criteria, or one major and three minor criteria, or five minor criteria. These are summarized as follows (Habib et al., 2015):

## Major Criteria

1. Positive blood cultures consistent with infective endocarditis
2. Echocardiogram demonstrating:
   a. Vegetation in the absence of an alternative explanation
   b. Abscess
   c. New or partial dehiscence of a prosthetic valve

## Minor Criteria

1. Predisposition such as a underlying heart condition or intravenous drug use
2. Fever
3. Vascular phenomenon (septic emboli)
4. Immunological phenomena—glomerulonephritis, Osler's nodes, Roth spots, and rheumatoid factor
5. Microbiological evidence (positive blood cultures but not meeting major criteria)
6. Echocardiogram findings but not meeting major criteria

**Likely Diagnosis:** Infective endocarditis

---

### WHAT'S NEXT?

The resolution of this case was described earlier. The patient required lengthy inpatient treatment and was eventually discharged with normalized cardiac function.

---

# SUMMARIZING THE SCENARIO

This case scenario provided another presentation in which positive troponin values were not indicative of an MI. The levels were elevated but remained fairly flat, without the typical rise-and-fall pattern seen in an MI.

This patient had months of symptoms that were suggestive of a malignancy or ongoing infection. The identification of the murmur on exam narrowed the differential down to a likely cause of endocarditis. The imaging tests demonstrated the presence of septic emboli, both in the brain and in the spleen, further supporting a likely cardiac origin. The echocardiogram and TEE confirmed the vegetation on the aortic valve, which resulted in the severe aortic insufficiency that prompted emergent surgical correction.

This patient had infective endocarditis and anemia that further propagated the potential to have abnormal troponin levels. We have discussed how these levels can be abnormal in endocarditis as well as in sepsis and anemia. This patient had multiple contributory issues, any of which in isolation could have resulted in an elevated troponin level. It seems reasonable to assume that troponin levels would be anything but normal in this case scenario.

## COMMON PITFALLS AND ASSUMPTIONS

Nurse practitioners, physician assistants, and physicians who specialize in cardiology may feel that troponins are the bane of their existence. Consults for elevated troponin levels constitute much of their work in the acute care setting. When these abnormalities occur, cardiovascular clinicians are called upon to lend their expertise in identifying a cause, determining significance, and outlining the best course of action.

It is important to consider how useful any testing or laboratory data will be to the treatment course of the patient in a given clinical context. Clinicians often react instinctively by checking troponin levels when a patient develops hemodynamic instability and worsening changes on ECG. In most cases it is not necessarily wrong to order the test, but one should still question whether the information obtained will change management. If management will not change regardless of the result, then perhaps the need for the test should be reconsidered.

It is common for troponin levels to be elevated in patients with a critical illness, such as sepsis or endocarditis, and in the presence of gastrointestinal bleeding. In these instances, the troponin elevation indicates a worse prognosis rather than the presence of obstructive coronary artery disease. Troponin elevation is associated with an increased risk of death in sepsis (Sheyin et al., 2015) and a worse prognosis in endocarditis (Thoker et al., 2016).

As we saw in Chapter 7, differentiating between type I and type II MI can be quite difficult, particularly in postoperative patients, in those with renal disease or heart failure, and in the critically ill. Often there are supply-and-demand issues in the postoperative period due to alterations in heart rate and blood pressure, or bleeding. Likewise, trying to evaluate for ischemic symptoms in a critically ill patient who is intubated and sedated becomes challenging, but this symptom evaluation is necessary in order to diagnose an MI.

Recently, newer, high-sensitivity troponin assays have been approved for use in the United States. As a result, we can expect to see increasing instances of troponin release reported in non-MI situations. As cardiovascular clinicians, we must understand all the various mechanisms for troponin release and their relevance in a given case scenario. Troponin elevation does not always equate with myocardial injury, and it is important that the clinician not be distracted by this objective piece of data, but rather correlate it with the clinical context in order to narrow the differential.

# REFERENCES

Baddour, L., Freeman, W., Rakesh, M., Wilson, S., & Wilson, W. (2015). Cardiovascular infections. In D. L. Mann, D. P. Zipes, P. Libby, & R. O. Bonow *Braunwald's heart disease: A textbook of cardiovascular medicine* (10th ed., 1524–1550). Philadelphia, PA: Elsevier/Saunders.

Habib, G., Lancellotti, P., Antunes, M., Bongiorni, M., Casalta, J., Del Zotti, F., … Zamorano, J. (2015). ESC Guidelines for the management of infective endocarditis: The task force for the management of infective endocartitis of the ESC.

Januzzi Jr., J. (2010). Causes of non-ACS related troponin elevations. *American College of Cardiology.* Retrieved from http://www.acc.org/latest-in-cardiology/articles/2014/07/18/13/16/causes-of-non-acs-related-troponin-elevations

Sheyin, O., Davies, O., Duan, W., & Perez, X. (2015). The prognostic significance of troponin elevation in patients with sepsis: A meta-analysis. *Heart & Lung: The Journal of Acute and Critical Care, 44*(1), 75–81.

Tettamanti, C., Hervet, T., Grabherr, S., & Palmeire, C. (2016). Elevation of NT-proBNP and cardiac troponins in sepsis -related deaths: A forensic perspective. *International Journal of Legal Medicine, 130*(4), 1035–1043.

Thoker, Z., Khan, K., Rashid, I., & Zafar. (2016). Correlation of cardiac troponin I levels with infective endocarditis & its adverse clinical outcomes. *International Journal of Cardiology, 222,* 661–664. doi:10.1016/j.ijcard.2016.07.13

Wan, S., Liang, J., Vaidya, R., Blackshear, J., & Chen, D. (2014). Acquired Von Willebrand syndrome secondary to mitral and aortic regurgitation. *Canadian Journal of Cardiology, 30*(9), 1108.e9–1108.e10. doi:10.1016/j.cjca.2014.02.010

# PART II

# Uncommon Presentations of Acute Cardiac Conditions

In Part I of this book, we looked at many different case scenarios with primary symptoms that are often present in acute cardiac conditions. We learned that despite the initial presentation, many of those symptoms do not always result from a primary cardiac diagnosis. In other instances, we discovered that the chief complaint did represent a cardiac condition, just not the one that was initially suspected.

As cardiovascular clinicians, when we encounter a patient experiencing syncope, shortness of breath, or chest discomfort of any kind, we immediately scan a mental list of differential diagnoses to determine if the case presentation is an acute cardiac condition. As we have learned from this book so far, things are not always what they seem. Often, common presentations with common symptoms lead to an expected diagnosis. Other times, common presentations with common symptoms lead to an unexpected diagnosis. And occasionally, uncommon presentations with common symptoms lead to an unexpected diagnosis—confronting the health care provider with a challenging dilemma.

We all face the "unusual" patient case from time to time—a clinical scenario that leaves us in awe and wonderment as to how a certain diagnosis was derived from such an atypical presentation. Often, these rare presentations are written up in journals so others can learn from them and remain alert, in their own practices, to the possibility that these rare circumstances can occur.

In Chapters 9, 10, and 11, we discuss uncommon presentations of acute cardiac conditions in patient with fatigue, cough, and abdominal pain. These are cases in which a vague chief complaint turns out to be something unexpected. The intent is to demonstrate how differences in the history can give clues to an alternate diagnosis in much the same manner that has been shown thus far. Rather than presenting two clinical scenarios for each chief complaint, as was done in Part I, we review one example of each presentation, due to the atypical nature of the cases.

# CHAPTER 9

# Fatigue

## DEFINITION AND SIGNIFICANCE OF FATIGUE

According to *Farlex Medical Dictionary* (2012), fatigue is "that state, following a period of mental or bodily activity, characterized by a lessened capacity for work and reduced efficiency of accomplishment, usually accompanied by a feeling of weariness, sleepiness or irritability; may also supervene when, from any cause, energy expenditure outstrips restorative processes and may be confined to a single organ."

Fatigue is a very broad and general symptom that can be present in a host of diseases. It is often coupled with other complaints that help to identify the primary underlying process. It is present in healthy and nonhealthy individuals alike, and there is no one event that causes it, making it even more challenging to quantify in the healthcare setting. When there is an underlying illness, fatigue is rarely present in isolation as the sole symptom. This may not, however, be obvious initially to the patient or the provider until a deep and comprehensive history is taken.

Most people do not seek acute medical attention for fatigue. They may report the symptom to their primary care physician or may dismiss it as a natural part of growing older or being out of shape. However, fatigue can be representative of a serious underlying condition, and it is important to stress to patients that prolonged symptoms of fatigue, despite adequate rest, nutrition, and perceived health should not be ignored.

What defines a "classic presentation" of any disease is the frequency with which particular symptoms are seen and the physiological process of the disease that produces those symptoms. Nonetheless, many individuals do not present with typical symptoms. This situation can lead to a delay either in seeking medical attention or in identifying a diagnosis, thus increasing the possibility of negative outcomes.

Fatigue may be present in many cardiovascular conditions. Again, it is usually part of a greater constellation of symptoms, but this is not always the case. Clinicians must consider the population in which atypical symptoms are more likely to be present, keep an open mind, and not be too quick to dismiss symptoms of fatigue without ensuring that we are evaluating for an acute underlying condition if the clinical picture calls for it.

A case scenario for a patient with a presenting complaint of fatigue follows. As in earlier chapters, let us explore how the initial history taken by an emergency physician contrasts with that obtained by a consulting cardiovascular clinician. Pay particular attention to how variances in the history-taking process can change the details obtained, and thus the course of treatment.

## CASE SCENARIO

A 76-year-old White female is brought into the emergency department with a chief complaint of fatigue and decreased energy. Her daughter states that she went to check on her mother today and found her in bed, reporting an inability to get up and get dressed due to her fatigue. Her daughter was concerned as this behavior is out of character for her mother; therefore, she brought her mother in for evaluation. The initial blood pressure reading is 110/78 mmHg, pulse is 51 beats per minute, respiratory rate is 16 breaths per minute, and oxygen saturation is 97% on room air. She is afebrile.

The emergency physician asks the patient the following questions to obtain a history:

Q: **Can you tell me why you came in to the emergency department today?**

A: I have been really tired with no energy lately.

Q: **How long has this been going on?**

    A: Several weeks. I thought I had a virus and didn't think much of it, but I just can't seem to get better.

Q: **Do you remember when you first noticed it and what you were doing?**

    A: About 3 weeks ago I guess. I came home after running errands and I felt I had to take a nap, which I never do. But now I am always tired, although I nap during the day and sleep okay at night. I just feel "zapped."

Q: **Did the symptoms start gradually or did they seem to begin all of a sudden?**

    A: Gradually.

Q: **Does anything make the feeling better or worse?**

    A: Not really.

Q: **Do you have any chest pain, pressure, or shortness of breath?**

    A: No. I'm just really tired.

Q: **Have you had any dizziness, lightheadedness, or fainting?**

    A: No, but I really haven't done very much in a while.

Q: **Have you noticed any palpitations or abnormal heart beats?**

    A: No.

Q: **Have there been any changes in your medications recently?**

    A: No. I've been on the same medications for years.

Q: **Any recent illnesses or travel?**

    A: No.

Q: **Have you noticed any dark or tarry stools, or any changes to your bowel or bladder patterns?**

    A: No.

Q: **Has there been any change in your appetite or weight?**

    A: No. I watch my diet very carefully. I eat the same things pretty religiously.

Q: **Have you traveled anywhere recently?**

    A: No. I went on a cruise 3 months ago, but nothing since.

Q: Do you smoke or drink, or take any over-the-counter medications or use drugs?

A: I smoked for about 15 years but quit 40 years ago. I have a glass of wine occasionally but haven't had a drink since this started, and I don't take anything but Tylenol on occasion for a headache.

Q: Do you have any history of thyroid problems, cancer, or heart problems?

A: I have high blood pressure and I take valsartan, 80 mg daily. Other than that I've been healthy.

Initial laboratory data reveal a normal complete blood count (CBC) with differential, normal chemistry panel, and normal thyroid-stimulating hormone (TSH) level. Liver function studies are also normal. A chest film is negative for any fluid or infectious or inflammatory process. A brain natriuretic peptide (BNP) test is normal, and troponin T is undetectable at less than 0.01 ng/mL. An ECG shows Mobitz type I second-degree atrioventricular (AV) block, with a rate of 49 beats per minute and non-specific T-wave flattening in lead aVL. The physical exam performed by the emergency physician is unremarkable for any findings. Given the second-degree heart block seen on the ECG, a cardiology consult is arranged to determine whether the heart block could be the cause of the patient's fatigue.

The emergency physician summarizes the patient's presentation (history A) to the consulting cardiovascular clinician.

# HISTORY A

*A 76-year-old White female with a past medical history of hypertension presented to the emergency department today with a 3-week history of profound fatigue and decreased energy. She perceives the symptoms as starting gradually with fatigue that required a nap after running errands. She states she does not usually nap during the day and has been getting adequate sleep at night; however, she feels "zapped" all the time. She initially thought she had a virus of some kind, but the symptoms have progressed to the point of her having difficulty getting out of bed this morning to get dressed, prompting her daughter to bring her in for evaluation.*

*She has had no changes in her medications and no recent bleeding, weight loss, or changes in appetite. She denies any other associated symptoms such as chest pain, palpitations, dizziness, near syncope, or shortness of breath. Her exam and laboratory data are unremarkable. However, her ECG reveals Mobitz type I second-degree AV block. We are concerned her fatigue may be due to this condition and we would like cardiology's recommendations for further management.*

The cardiovascular clinician reviews the patient's chart and relevant data. A prior ECG in the hospital database from 6 months ago shows normal sinus rhythm with a heart rate of 62 beats per minute. As the cardiovascular clinician arrives to the emergency department, the following vital signs are obtained from the patient. The cardiovascular clinician obtains:

*Blood pressure*: Right arm, 114/68 mmHg; left arm, 114/72 mmHg

*Pulse*: 48 to 54 beats per minute

*Respirations*: 14 breaths per minute

*Oxygen saturation*: 97% on room air

*Temperature*: 36.7°C

The clinician asks the patient the following questions:

Q: **What brought you to the emergency department today?**

A: I have been feeling really tired with no energy for a few weeks. I could hardly get out of bed today when my daughter checked on me, so she brought me in.

Q: **Have you ever felt this way before?**

A: No.

Q: **Do you notice anything that makes you feel more fatigued or lessens the fatigue?**

A: No.

Q: **Are you having any other symptoms such as chest pain or discomfort, arm pain, back pain, jaw pain, or shortness of breath?**

A: No. I haven't noticed anything like that.

Q: Have you felt dizzy or lightheaded—like you were going to pass out—or have you passed out?

A: No.

Q: Have you had any headaches, blurred vision, changes in your thinking, or weakness?

A: No, none of that.

Q: Have you had any abdominal pain or abnormal vaginal bleeding?

A: No.

Q: Have you noticed any bleeding in your stool or urine, changes in your bowel or bladder patterns, or nausea or vomiting?

A: No.

Q: Have you had any excessively dry or sweaty skin or any hair loss?

A: No.

Q: What were you doing when you first noticed the symptoms?

A: I remember about 3 weeks ago I was out running errands. When I came home I was extremely tired, which is unusual for me. I'm very active. But I took a nap that day.

Q: Were you experiencing any fevers, chills, or had you been around anyone sick?

A: No. I did think it was a virus initially, but it has hung around and progressed to the point that I feel really drained all the time.

Q: Did you see your doctor or call him at any time for these symptoms?

A: No.

Q: Do you feel that your symptoms have progressed gradually or was there any point in the past 3 weeks you feel that the fatigue got profoundly worse?

A: It has been gradual, but these past few days have been the worst. I've had trouble just doing the day-to-day activities without feeling tired and needing to take a break.

Q: **How active were you on a daily basis prior to feeling this way? Did you exercise?**

A: I am always on the go. You can ask anyone who knows me. I volunteer a lot and I take Zumba twice a week and walk with my neighbors three times a week for about 2 miles. But I haven't been able to do any of that in about 2 weeks.

Q: **Are you normally able to exercise and do this kind of activity without experiencing any shortness of breath, chest discomfort, or fatigue?**

A: Absolutely! In fact, I typically have more energy after doing these things. I tried to go to my Zumba class after about a week of feeling this way, but I had to leave. I just couldn't do any of it.

Q: **Have you been sleeping well at night or are there any significant stressors right now in your life?**

A: I have slept too well and too long at night for the past few weeks. I do not feel stressed at all, just frustrated that I have no energy.

Q: **Do you have any other medical history besides high blood pressure? Do you have any thyroid problems, cancer, diabetes, heart problems, or lung problems?**

A: No. I have been really lucky. I don't really get sick.

Q: **Do you follow up regularly with your primary care doctor?**

A: Yes. I get my annual checkups. I just saw him 6 months ago.

Q: **How is your appetite? Have there been any changes to your diet?**

A: I eat the same things each day for the most part. I'm very health conscious and watch what I eat closely. My appetite hasn't changed.

Q: **Have any of your medications changed recently?**

A: No. I'm on valsartan, 80 mg daily, and I take a baby aspirin daily.

Q: **Do you smoke or drink or have you ever?**

A: I smoked a little for 15 years. I quit 40 years ago. I drink an occasional glass of wine, but have not had any in 3 weeks.

**Q: Do you use any illicit drugs or over-the-counter medications?**

A: No, never. I take an occasional Tylenol for pain if I need it.

**Q: Have you ever been told you have a low heart rate?**

A: My heart rate is usually in the 60s. I've never been told it is a problem.

**Q: Do you ever notice what your heart rate does when you exercise?**

A: No. I don't pay attention.

**Q: Have you ever had a stress test before or any other kind of cardiac test such as a heart catheterization or echocardiogram?**

A: I think I may have had an echocardiogram years ago, but I don't recall the reason.

The cardiovascular clinician performs an exam, which is detailed later, and summarizes the patient's presenting complaint as follows.

# HISTORY B

*A 76-year-old White female with a past medical history only of hypertension presented to the emergency department today with a 3-week history of fatigue and decreased energy. She initially noticed the symptoms after running errands one day and felt the need to rest and take a nap, which is unusual for her. She denies any associated infectious symptoms at that time, but did perceive it to be a virus although she did not seek medical attention. She is normally quite active and takes Zumba classes along with frequent 2-mile walks without having any negative symptoms. However, she noted about 2 weeks ago that she could no longer complete her Zumba class due to her fatigue.*

*She feels that the fatigue has been gradual in onset, but notes that it has been more profound over the past few days, resulting in a loss of energy that is affecting her activities of daily living. This situation ultimately prompted her daughter to bring her in for evaluation.*

*She denies experiencing any chest pain or discomfort or any shortness of breath. She has no jaw pain, back pain, or arm pain. She denies any dizziness, lightheadedness, syncope, or near syncope. She denies any abdominal pain, nausea, vomiting, or abnormal bleeding. She denies any headaches or neurological symptoms. She has had no major stressors and no changes in weight or appetite. Her hypertension is well controlled with medication that has not changed or been altered recently.*

Without considering any objective data and looking at only the history, what differentials are at the top of your list at this point? What needs to be done to further identify the cause of this patient's fatigue?

## KEY FEATURES OF THE HISTORY

In any patient with a chief complaint of fatigue, it is important that the history be extremely thorough. Fatigue can be representative of many conditions, and it is important to ask the right questions in order to thoroughly evaluate every system. We cannot assume that patients will disclose details on their own without being prompted by certain questions.

The emergency physician and the cardiovascular clinician asked very detailed questions about the patient's symptoms. As noted in previous chapters, the features of the history can often overlap. Let us compare the two histories and discuss the differences to see whether they change the differential.

### Character

The symptom of fatigue is very hard to characterize. Much like syncope, it does not localize and cannot be quantified by descriptive terms such as "sharp," "pressure," or "tightness," similar to the way we characterize chest pain.

Both providers identified that the patient was feeling fatigued and had decreased energy. The provider in history A was able to extract that the patient felt "zapped" and found herself taking more naps. The provider in history B also noted this information, but was able to further identify that the patient was very active at baseline and could no longer exercise as she had done previously due to her symptoms.

The cardiovascular clinician also identified that the patient's symptoms had worsened in severity within the past few days, which resulted in an inability to perform daily activities. This distinction is important, as her fatigue had not been at the same level for 3 weeks, but had worsened. This finding suggests that the underlying process that is occurring is becoming more profound or severe.

The patient told both providers that she felt she had a virus at the outset of experiencing the fatigue, but only the cardiovascular nurse practitioner questioned her further about this associated illness and whether she saw her primary care physician about it. It is always important to ask patients if and when they sought medical attention for symptoms prior to their current presentation. This information helps to establish a timeline and identify any treatment that may have been provided or prescribed for the illness.

## Timing and Duration

The emergency physician asked the patient when the symptoms started and how long they had been occurring. The cardiovascular clinician obtained the same information, and both providers learned that her symptoms were gradual in onset and were first noticed after she ran errands about 3 weeks ago. The cardiovascular clinician also established that she had never experienced these symptoms before and that they have worsened in the past week.

## Associated Symptoms

The emergency physician and the cardiovascular clinician asked about associated symptoms such as chest pain, palpitations, shortness of breath, dizziness, lightheadedness, syncope, or near syncope, as well as any changes in bowel or bladder patterns and bleeding. The cardiovascular clinician asked more comprehensive questions about associated symptoms, including abdominal symptoms, neurological symptoms, vaginal bleeding, hair loss, and skin changes. Why do you think these questions were asked?

Since fatigue can be a symptom of almost any disease, these questions were asked to determine whether the patient was having any symptoms suggestive of thyroid problems or malignancy. The patient had voiced no other associated symptoms to help narrow down the search, so it was important to ask detailed questions about each system, specifically to avoid overlooking a subtle sign or abnormality that might otherwise go unnoticed. For instance, if she had had minor vaginal bleeding or spotting, she might not have thought to offer this information or have seen its relevance until asked specifically about it, yet this can be a sign of uterine cancer, which often has no symptoms initially except perhaps bleeding or fatigue. With such a broad symptom as fatigue, these types of questions can be critical to making the right diagnosis.

## Mitigating or Alleviating Factors

In this clinical scenario, there were no factors that made the patient's fatigue better or worse. She reported to both providers that, although she had been getting adequate rest, she did not have the energy to do anything. The cardiovascular clinician focused more deeply on the patient's baseline activity. The fact she could no longer make it through her Zumba class when she had until recently been able to do so without any difficulty showed a significant decline in functional status. This relevant piece of data is explored in more detail when we discuss the differential diagnoses a bit later in the chapter. Since the cause of fatigue can be multifactorial, the cardiovascular clinician also asked the patient about stress, and both providers questioned her about appetite as well as medication or dietary changes.

# KEY FEATURES OF THE DATA

It is very difficult to know what laboratory and diagnostic tests to order when a patient presents with a complaint of fatigue and decreased energy. As is true in any clinical case, the diagnostic tests, as well as baseline vital signs, ECG, and imaging studies, can help in identifying a cause or eliminating it. Let us take a closer look.

## Vital Signs

Recall that the following findings were obtained by the cardiovascular clinician:

*Blood pressure*: Right arm, 114/68 mmHg; left arm, 114/72 mmHg

*Pulse*: 48 to 54 beats per minute

*Respirations*: 14 breaths per minute

*Oxygen saturation*: 97% on room air

*Temperature*: 36.7°C

The patient is obviously bradycardic; however, we learned that her baseline heart rate is usuaclly in the 60s, so these readings are not considerably lower than her baseline. Is her current heart rate enough to cause her symptoms?

## Electrocardiogram (ECG)

The ECG was carefully reviewed and notable for Mobitz type I second-degree AV block. There was T-wave flattening in leads I and aVL. These findings were not present on an ECG obtained 6 months ago.

## Chest Radiograph

The chest film did not demonstrate any findings consistent with heart failure, lung disease, pneumonia, or any other abnormalities. The mediastinum and heart size were within normal limits.

## Biomarkers and Lab Results

If a patient presents with fatigue, it is important to evaluate for any anemia, electrolyte disturbances, and thyroid problems. The patient's laboratory data did not lend any clues to her underlying issue. Laboratory studies are performed. Her CBC with differential, chemistry panel, TSH, BNP, troponin T level, and liver function studies were within normal limits. Therefore, anemia, infection, or metabolic processes are likely not contributing to her symptoms.

## Other Data

The patient's medications were reviewed throughout the evaluation and were notable only for valsartan, 80 mg daily, and aspirin, 81 mg daily, as well as daily calcium and vitamin supplements. She occasionally takes Tylenol for pain but is otherwise on no other medications.

The pertinent medical history was notable only for hypertension. The patient indicated that she follows up regularly with her primary care provider. Additionally, she has had no major surgeries other than one cesarean section. She has a remote smoking history with occasional alcohol use. When asked about family history, she reports that her father had prostate cancer and her mother had hypertension and lived to be 98 years of age.

# DIFFERENTIALS AND DIFFERENCES IN EXAM

The initial exam performed by the emergency physician was unremarkable for any significant findings that would explain the patient's symptoms of fatigue. After the history is taken, the cardiovascular clinician examines the patient and notes the following findings:

*General appearance: Well-nourished, fit White female who appears younger than stated age and is not in acute distress.*

*Head and neck: Head is normocephalic and atraumatic, without evidence of lesions or masses. Sclera are anicteric. Neck is soft and supple, without thyromegaly or lymphadenopathy.*

*Cardiac exam: No elevation of jugular venous pressure. No carotid bruits. No femoral or abdominal bruits. Carotid upstrokes are symmetric and brisk. Peripheral pulses are palpable and symmetric. Auscultation of the heart reveals a regular rate and rhythm, S1 and S2 present. No S3 or S4. No murmurs or rubs. Chest wall is nontender to palpation.*

*Lungs: Clear breath sounds in bilateral lung fields with symmetric expansion.*

*Abdomen: Obese. Nontender. Bowel sounds present in all four quadrants. No hepatosplenomegaly. No hepatojugular reflux.*

*Extremities: Warm and dry. No edema, clubbing, or cyanosis.*

*Neurological: Alert and oriented ×3. Cranial nerves are intact. Motor strength is symmetric in bilateral upper and lower extremities. No focal neurological deficits.*

The physical exam was normal without any suspicious findings. Do you have any clues as to what could be going on in this case? Do you think this patient's fatigue is from her second-degree heart block or do you now think it is something else? Do we need more information?

At this point, the cardiovascular clinician has some thoughts as to the cause of the patient's fatigue and how to proceed. It is unlikely that Mobitz type I second-degree AV block would cause such profound fatigue. Let us review the differential diagnoses for a chief complaint of fatigue, categorized by system. Since this list is very broad, we will break it down by system.

# PULLING IT ALL TOGETHER

## Working Through the Differential

There are many diseases within each system that can cause fatigue and decreased energy. We need to consider the clinical context and any other associated symptoms so we can ideally narrow the focus to one system.

**Differential Diagnoses of Fatigue—Systems Considered (*see text discussion*)**

- Cardiac
- Malignancy
- Mental health
- Metabolic
- Neurological
- Pulmonary
- Rheumatological
- Infectious

COPD, chronic obstructive pulmonary disease; PAH, pulmonary arterial hypertension

Is there anything about this clinical scenario that would lead you to believe there is an infectious etiology at play? It appears that we can eliminate this as a contributing factor.

- The patient had no fever.
- No evidence of leukocytosis was detected.
- Chest film is without any infectious etiology.
- No other clinical signs and symptoms of infection are present, although it would not be unreasonable to check a urinalysis to be thorough.

What about any metabolic disorders, such as diabetes, thyroid problems, liver and kidney abnormalities, or malnutrition? These disorders are an unlikely source of her fatigue.

- She was not diabetic, as her glucose in the chemistry panel was normal.
- Her TSH was normal; however, further thyroid studies such as a free T4 and T3 would not be unreasonable.
- Liver function and kidney function were normal.
- She had a good appetite and is of adequate weight without reports of weight loss.
- She does not exhibit any clinical signs of poor nutrition.

Malignancy is always a concern when someone presents with fatigue. It is unusual for a malignancy to present with this solitary symptom; however, many other symptoms that might be present and indicative of cancer may be dismissed by the patient or ignored.

The history included questions regarding possible signs of malignancy, such as abnormal bleeding, weight loss, and changes in appetite. The patient denied all of these symptoms. Although she was not questioned about any abnormal findings on breast exam, it would not have been unreasonable to inquire about this aspect as well. As she stated that she has annual physical exams, you can assume she is up to date on her preventative cancer screening. According to the thorough history obtained, she has given no clues that there may be an underlying malignant process; therefore, we can likely eliminate this diagnosis from our list.

Depression and anxiety as well as physical or emotional stress can certainly produce fatigue and lack of energy disproportionate to the activity. This patient denied any recent stressors and has no history of depression or anxiety. She did admit to being frustrated about her current state, but it does not appear that her mood or any mental health issues precipitated her symptoms.

Rheumatological disorders include Lyme disease, lupus, fibromyalgia, arthritis, and chronic fatigue syndrome. Many of these disorders require more extensive investigation with laboratory data and testing. These illnesses can cause fatigue, but are less probable.

- The patient had no joint pain, deformity, or history of arthritis.
- No physical manifestations were present, such as fever, joint pain, swelling, or rash.

The patient was asked about headaches, vision changes, changes in mentation, and weakness. She denied all of these symptoms. She is neurologically intact on exam without any focal neurological deficits and no symptoms of an underlying neurological process. Several neurological disorders are associated with severe fatigue and loss of energy, including multiple sclerosis. However, usually physical manifestations are associated with these conditions that are not present in this case. Therefore, an underlying neurological condition is less likely.

A primary pulmonary process is likely not the cause of the patient's fatigue.

- She had no cough or shortness of breath.
- A chest film was negative for any abnormal findings.
- The clinical exam was without evidence of pulmonary abnormality.

Cardiac conditions that cause fatigue can include myocardial ischemia, cardiomyopathies, heart failure, valvular disease, arrhythmias, conduction abnormalities, and infiltrative processes. Although the cardiovascular clinician was initially asked whether Mobitz type I second-degree AV block was precipitating the patient's fatigue, this is unlikely. This type of heart block rarely produces symptoms and, if it does, the symptoms are usually lightheadedness, dizziness, and syncope (Sovari, 2017). In this case, the AV block might be a manifestation of a more acute process.

An echocardiogram is needed to confirm the presence of any cardiomyopathy or valvular abnormality, but the patient had a normal cardiac exam without any murmurs or cardiomegaly noted.

Is it possible that this patient could be experiencing symptoms of cardiac ischemia? Advanced age increases the risk of cardiovascular disease. She also has hypertension, which is another risk factor. Although she smoked in the past, she has abstained for 40 years, which places her risk of coronary artery disease from tobacco use equal to that of a nonsmoker.

Atypical symptoms, or what most perceive to be "angina equivalents," are more likely to occur in the elderly and in women especially (Morrow & Boden, 2015). These symptoms include dyspnea, fatigue, decreased functional capacity, and faintness. Canto and colleagues reviewed common presenting symptoms of acute coronary symptoms in women and found that they were more likely than not to present without chest pain (Canto, Canto, & Goldberg, 2014). Knowing that this patient is at risk of having underlying heart disease, how does her second-degree Mobitz type I AV block fit into the picture if we are considering that ischemia is the cause of her fatigue?

In most individuals, the right coronary artery (RCA) supplies both the sinoatrial and the AV nodes (Assadi, 2016). If there is ischemia in the RCA, it can produce conduction system disturbances at any level and produce various degrees of AV block (Mega & Morrow, 2015). Advanced age alone can produce conduction system disturbances; however, in cases where the degree of AV block is disproportionate to the symptoms, ischemia of the RCA should be considered.

Although this patient's ECG did not demonstrate overt signs of ischemia, she did have T-wave flattening in leads I and aVL, which can be early signs of ischemia in the right clinical context and represent distal RCA disease (Mirvis & Goldberger, 2015). Both first-degree and second-degree heart block can be a common presentation in RCA ischemia. Therefore, in this case scenario, the focus should be on evaluating possible underlying myocardial ischemia as the cause of her fatigue.

**Likely Diagnosis**: Myocardial ischemia

---

WHAT'S NEXT?

- Based on the clinical suspicion of ischemia, the cardiovascular clinician orders an exercise echocardiogram stress test. The test demonstrates chronotropic incompetence with profound ST depression in lead aVL with inferior hypokinesis at peak exercise, which is highly suggestive of an RCA occlusion (Anjos-Andrade et al., 2010).

- The patient is taken for coronary angiography, which reveals mild disease throughout and a high-grade lesion in her distal RCA.

- She receives a drug-eluting stent to this region and is placed on ticagrelor, 90 mg twice daily, and continued on aspirin, 81 mg daily. No beta-blocker is initiated due to her slow heart rate.

- An echocardiogram performed shortly after this treatment shows preserved left and right ventricular function with an ejection fraction of 55%.

- A postreperfusion ECG demonstrates sinus rhythm with a heart rate of 62 beats per minute and resolution of the Mobitz type I second-degree AV block.

---

## SUMMARIZING THE SCENARIO

Fatigue in isolation of any other symptoms is an atypical presentation of ischemia; however, it should be considered as one of the top differential diagnoses particularly in elderly women. The presence of second-degree heart block further supports this rationale and should be considered as an additional sign and not a causative mechanism of her primary symptom.

Although heart block can produce symptoms, first-degree and second-degree Mobitz type I are unlikely to cause profound fatigue and marked decline in functional capacity. Many patients can become symptomatic from these conduction disturbances, especially when the heart rate has deviated a significant degree from their baseline. In this clinical scenario, we learned that the patient's normal heart rate was around 60 beats per minute, so a reduction to 40 to 50 beats per minute was unlikely to cause this degree of symptoms.

It may be instinctual in these cases to consider supporting the conduction system abnormality with various modalities, such as temporary pacing and electrophysiological study, but specific therapy is usually not required in this setting as long as the heart rate remains greater than 50 beats per minute consistently (Mega & Morrow, 2015). However, it would not be unreasonable to initiate these procedures in cases of advanced heart block, to provide for hemodynamic support and prevent further deterioration of the patient's clinical condition.

This case is an excellent example of how providers can become sidetracked by objective data, thus failing to consider whether the clinical presentation is truly a cause or consequence of the chief complaint. The cardiovascular clinician asked more detailed questions about the patient's baseline functional status and was able to clearly identify the significant change in it, which supported the suspicion of a potential ischemic cause for her fatigue.

It is always important to look at the entire clinical picture and consider the impact of the objective data when determining the best course of action. Patients do not always present with classic findings and, as cardiovascular clinicians, we must always be thinking about the uncommon and rare manifestations of acute cardiac conditions.

# REFERENCES

Anjos-Andrade, F., Sousa, A., Barreto-Filho, J., Alves, E., Nascimento-Júnior, A., De Santana, N., … Oliveira, J. (2010). Chronotropic incompetence and coronary artery disease. *Acta Cardiology*, 65(6), 631–638.

Assadi, R. (2016). *Conduction system of the heart*. Retrieved from http://www.emedicine.medscape.com/article/1922987-overview#a2

Canto, J., Canto, E., & Goldberg, R. (2014). Time to standardize and broaden the criteria of acute coronary syndrome symptom presentations in women. *Canadian Journal of Cardiology, 30*(2014), 721–728.

Farlex Medical Dictionary. (2012). Fatigue. Retrieved from http://medical-dictionary.thefreedictionary.com/fatigue

Mega, J., & Morrow, D. (2015). ST-Elevation myocardial infarction: Management. In D. L. Mann, D. P. Zipes, P. Libby, & R. O. Bonox, *Braunwald's heart disease: A textbook of cardiovascular medicine* (10th ed., pp. 1095–1154). Philadelphia, PA: Elsevier/Saunders.

Mirvis, D., & Goldberger, A. (2015). Electrocardiographic localization of myocardial ischemia and infarction. In D. L. Mann, D. P. Zipes, P. Libby, & R. O. Bonox, *Braunwald's heart disease: A textbook of cardiovascular medicine* (10th ed., 114–154). Philadelphia, PA: Elsevier/Saunders.

Morrow, D., & Boden, W. (2015). Stable ischemic heart disease. In D. L. Mann, D.P. Zipes, P. Libby, & R. O. Bonox, *Braunwald's heart disease: A textbook of cardiovascular medicine* (10th ed., 1182–1244). Philadelphia, PA: Elsevier/Saunders.

Sovari, A. (2017). Second-degree atrioventricular block. Retrieved from http://www.emedicine.medscape.com/article/161919-overview

# CHAPTER 10

# Cough

## DEFINITION AND CLINICAL SIGNFICANCE OF COUGH

Cough is defined by *Collins English Dictionary* (2014) as the following: "to expel air or solid matter from the lungs abruptly and explosively through the partially closed vocal chords." It is another very common complaint that can be representative of a multitude of conditions. According to the most recent National Hospital Ambulatory Medical Care Survey in 2013, a chief complaint of cough represented around 5 million visits to the emergency department per year (Rui, Kang, & Albert, 2013).

The presence of a cough is typically a response to some underlying lung process. This can be secondary to another mechanism that in turn affects the lungs, or the lungs themselves might be the primary source. Cough can be accompanied by other symptoms or it can be present in isolation as the primary chief complaint, just like fatigue. A primary symptom of cough, however, does not seem like a reason for most people to seek urgent medical attention. Most individuals would see their primary care physician first, depending on the associated factors. Although cough represents a significant reason for emergency department visits annually, as stated previously, these visits may represent patients who had already gone to their primary care provider, patients who did not have a primary care provider, or patients with symptoms that persisted despite treatment.

Individuals may delay seeking treatment for cough altogether, depending on the circumstances. The cough may be seen as merely a nuisance and not representative of an acute process, or it may be blamed on environmental factors such as allergies or irritants. The presence of a cough, however, can be an indicator of a significant problem, and its persistence should not be ignored or dismissed.

The history is the most critical piece of information when evaluating a patient with cough. Any associated symptoms, the presence or absence of phlegm, and any mitigating factors are key in determining the cause of and ultimately the treatment for the cough.

Let us review a case scenario to demonstrate this concept.

## CASE SCENARIO

An 80-year-old White male presents to the emergency department with a complaint of cough. Initial vital signs are as follows: blood pressure, 165/82 mmHg; pulse, 76 beats per minute; respiratory rate, 18 breaths per minute; oxygen saturation, 95% on room air; and temperature, 36.6°C.

The emergency physician asks the following questions to learn more about his chief complaint:

**Q: Why did you come to the emergency department today?**

A: I have this hacking cough that won't go away.

**Q: When did the cough start?**

A: About a month ago, I guess.

**Q: Were you sick at the time? Any fevers?**

A: No, nothing like that. I noticed that I was starting to cough a little more than usual for no apparent reason.

**Q: Was the cough productive or is it productive now?**

A: No. That's the difference from my usual cough. It seems to be dry and hacking. Once in a while I cough up some phlegm, but that is normal for me with my chronic obstructive pulmonary disease (COPD).

**Q: Is the sputum clear in color or not?**

A: Thick and white, if at all. Like I said, that is normal for me.

**Q: Did you take anything to help your cough?**

A: I tried using my inhaler, but it didn't seem to help.

Q: **Did you seek treatment when you first noticed it?**

A: I went to my family doctor after about 5 days and he treated me for a COPD flare-up.

Q: **Did you feel any improvement after that?**

A: Not really. I feel like each day has gotten worse and I haven't slept in days. I need some relief. I can't seem to do anything because I'm so tired from the cough.

Q: **Are you having any other symptoms such as shortness of breath, chest pain, dizziness, nausea, or vomiting?**

A: I live with a little shortness of breath, but I can't really tell that it is worse.

Q: **Are you short of breath at rest, or mainly with activity?**

A: If I'm up and about too long I get winded. I'm okay at rest.

Q: **Have you taken anything else over the counter for the cough?**

A: No.

Q: **Have any of your medications changed recently?**

A: No.

Q: **Any environmental allergies or allergies to medications?**

A: No.

Q: **Do you have a history of heart disease, cancer, or any lung problems aside from COPD?**

A: I have coronary artery disease and high blood pressure. I also have high cholesterol. I have never had cancer. I use a machine at night for sleep apnea.

Q: **How was your coronary artery disease diagnosed?**

A: I had a heart catheterization a few years back—had some minor blockages but didn't need any stents.

Q: **Have you ever had a blood clot to your lungs or your legs, or any heart rhythm problems?**

A: I have a history of atrial fibrillation and I take warfarin.

Q: **Do you have any thyroid problems, diabetes, or kidney problems?**

A: I am diabetic. I take metformin.

**Q: Any abnormal bleeding?**

A: No.

**Q: Do you smoke or drink?**

A: I smoked a lot in the Navy—a pack a day for about 30-plus years. I quit 25 years ago. I don't drink. Never did any drugs.

Baseline laboratory data are obtained, revealing a normal complete blood count (CBC) with a white blood cell (WBC) count on the upper limits of normal, a normal chemistry panel, and a troponin T level of less than 0.01 ng/mL. The international normalized ratio (INR) level is 2.2. An ECG is performed and it shows normal sinus rhythm, and no ST–T-wave abnormalities or signs of ischemia. A chest film shows bilateral pleural effusions with increased interstitial markings suggestive of pulmonary edema. A brain natriuretic peptide (BNP) level is then obtained, and the result is 269 ng/L.

The emergency physician performs a physical exam and notes morbid obesity with mild dependent edema in the patient's lower extremities. Lung sounds are notable for inspiratory and expiratory wheezing bilaterally. The cardiology service is then consulted for presumed mild heart failure exacerbation and asked for recommendations in management and possibly early discharge from the emergency department.

The emergency physician summarizes the patient's presentation to the consulting cardiovascular clinician as follows:

## HISTORY A

*An 80-year-old obese White male with a past medical history of hypertension, atrial fibrillation, hyperlipidemia, type 2 diabetes, coronary artery disease, obstructive sleep apnea, and COPD presented to the emergency department with a complaint of cough that is different from his baseline. The cough began around 1 month ago. He describes the cough as dry and hacking in nature, different from his usual semiproductive cough from his COPD. He denies any associated illness at the time or any fevers or chills. He initially used his inhaler to obtain relief, but it did not help. Therefore, he saw his family doctor after a week of symptoms. He was treated for a COPD exacerbation at that time.*

*He denies any associated symptoms such as shortness of breath or chest pain. He continues to feel poorly, with an inability to sleep due to his cough. Initial laboratory data are significant only for a slightly elevated WBC and a BNP of 269 pg/mL. Chest film is concerning for some pulmonary edema and pleural effusions, and he has wheezes in bilateral lung fields on exam with some depended edema. This appears to be a mild heart failure exacerbation and we would like cardiology's assistance in management.*

The cardiovascular clinician reviews the data and proceeds to evaluate the patient. Vital signs are repeated and are as follows:

*Blood pressure*: Left arm, 166/80 mmHg; right arm, 172/82 mmHg

*Pulse*: 78 beats per minute

*Respirations*: 16 breaths per minute

*Oxygen saturation*: 95% on room air

*Temperature*: 36.6°C

The cardiovascular clinician asks the patient the following questions:

**Q: What brings you to the emergency department today?**

A: I have this nagging cough that I can't get rid of.

**Q: How long has this been going on?**

A: For about a month.

**Q: When did you notice it coming on? What activity were you doing, or were you ill at the time?**

A: I have a cough now and again with my COPD. This was different though. I noticed it coming on one day but it was dry and hacking. Not like my usual COPD cough.

**Q: Were you doing anything in particular that you recall when you noticed it? Were you sleeping, or outside, or exercising?**

A: Come to think of it I was trying to take a nap and I seemed to cough more than usual.

**Q: Did you have any fevers or chills, or other symptoms of illness at the time?**

A: No, none at all.

Q: **Was your cough always dry and hacking or did you ever cough anything up? If so, what color was it?**

A: I cough up white phlegm often with my COPD. This was different. It was dry from the get go. It felt like a tickle I couldn't get rid of.

Q: **Did you have any shortness of breath or chest pain or chest discomfort or chest burning?**

A: No. I do tend to get short of breath if I'm up and about, but that has not changed in years.

Q: **Do you have any palpitations, nausea, vomiting, or back, arm, or jaw pain?**

A: No.

Q: **Have you coughed up any pink-tinged or bloody sputum at any time?**

A: No.

Q: **Do you have any abnormal bleeding from your bowels or any bleeding issues with warfarin?**

A: No.

Q: **Did you try and treat your cough initially at home with any medication?**

A: I took my inhaler, but it didn't help. So then I went to my family doctor.

Q: **How long had you been having the cough before you saw your family doctor?**

A: A week I think.

Q: **What did your doctor do?**

A: He thought it was a COPD exacerbation so he treated me for that.

Q: **Did you feel better at any point, or do you feel you are getting worse?**

A: I didn't really feel any improvement at all.

**Q: Is there any activity now that makes you cough more than another?**

A: Seems to be every time I lie down I cough. So, I've been getting up and sleeping in my recliner at night, but it's not very comfortable.

**Q: So, you cough more when you lie flat?**

A: I guess so. Yes.

**Q: Do you cough more when you eat, or is there any relationship with eating?**

A: No.

**Q: Have you noticed any changes in your activity or your ability to do activities since the cough began?**

A: Yes. I can hardly sleep because of the cough so I'm so tired during the day. I've been spending my time in my recliner watching TV and napping.

**Q: Have you noticed any changes in your weight or any swelling?**

A: Well I'm overweight, as you can see. I don't weigh myself because I know I need to lose it. I don't think my weight has changed. I haven't noticed any swelling.

**Q: Do you eat a lot of salt in your diet?**

A: No, hardly any. I don't add salt to anything. My daughter lives close by and helps out with cooking a lot. But she's been out of town for a few weeks and I've been eating those lean cuisine meals and soups.

**Q: I reviewed your chart and noticed you have a history of atrial fibrillation. How long ago was it diagnosed, and when was the last time you were in atrial fibrillation? Do you know?**

A: Oh, about 10 years, I'd say. I had a bout of atrial fibrillation about 2 years ago when I had pneumonia.

**Q: Can you tell when you are in atrial fibrillation? What are your symptoms?**

A: Sometimes I feel a little flutter in my chest or I will notice my heart rate to be higher when I check my blood pressure at home.

Q: Have you noticed any changes in your heart rate recently?

A: No.

Q: Have you had any dizziness, lightheadedness, fainting, or near fainting?

A: No

Q: Just to clarify, you have a history of high blood pressure, high cholesterol, diabetes, sleep apnea, and coronary artery disease as well?

A: Yes.

Q: Are you compliant with your continuous positive airway pressure (CPAP) machine?

A: Yes.

Q: Tell me how your coronary artery disease was diagnosed?

A: I had a heart catheterization a few years ago. But I didn't need any stents.

Q: Why was that done?

A: I was having a hernia repair and they did a stress test, which I guess didn't give a good result, so I had that other test. They said I had some blockages, but nothing bad enough for a stent.

Q: You used to smoke, correct? Do you drink or use any drugs?

A: I smoked for over 30 years, but I haven't had a cigarette in 25 years or so. I don't drink. Used to have my fair share in the Navy, but none now. I have never done any drugs.

Q: Have you ever been told you have a weakened heart muscle or that you've had a heart attack?

A: No.

Q: What does your blood pressure normally run at home?

A: It's usually in the 140s to 150s. It's been higher these past couple of weeks.

Q: Any changes to your medications recently or any allergies to anything?

A: No.

The cardiovascular clinician completes the exam and summarizes the history of present illness as follows.

## HISTORY B

*An 80-year-old obese White male with a past medical history of COPD, obstructive sleep apnea, coronary artery disease, atrial fibrillation, hypertension, hyperlipidemia, and diabetes mellitus type 2 presented to the emergency department today with a complaint of a dry, hacking cough that has been present for 1 month. The cough is nonproductive and differs from the occasional productive cough he experiences with his COPD. He denies any associated fevers or symptoms of illness. He initially used his inhaler but had no relief; therefore, he sought treatment from his family doctor after 1 week of symptoms. He was treated for a COPD exacerbation but never felt any improvement.*

*He states the cough comes on primarily when he is lying flat, requiring him to sleep in a recliner during the night for relief. He denies any other associated symptoms, such as shortness of breath that is worsened from his baseline, palpitations, chest pain, nausea, vomiting, or syncope or near syncope. He has not had any bleeding issues while taking warfarin for his atrial fibrillation.*

*Of note, he has had increased salt intake over the last few weeks in his daughter's absence with instant meals and soups. He denies any changes in weight or swelling but notes that his blood pressure has been elevated during this time frame as well. He has not noticed an increase in heart rate or symptoms consistent with his atrial fibrillation. He is compliant with his CPAP machine. He feels tired from his lack of sleep and spends the majority of his day sitting in his recliner.*

Does the preceding history paint a different picture than the first history summarized by the emergency physician? Without considering any objective data, can you make a presumptive diagnosis based on the history of present illness summarized in history A? Can you with history B? Let us discuss further.

## KEY FEATURES OF THE HISTORY

A chief complaint of cough requires a thorough and detailed history in order to narrow down potential causes. Cough can be caused by any number of things, including irritants, infections, underlying lung disease, malignancy, drug effect, heart failure, or reflux. To narrow this list, the events leading up to and surrounding the episodes of cough are crucial in determining the diagnosis. Let us review each key feature of the history and compare them again.

## Character

The emergency physician identified that the cough was dry, hacking, and for the most part nonproductive. The cardiovascular clinician acquired the same details. They both were able to determine that the patient's symptoms were more persistent, causing unrest, rather than increasing in severity. The patient provided helpful details by noting he had a cough intermittently at baseline, which he described as productive and associated with his COPD. He provided the distinctive detail that the current cough was different and new.

Had he not offered this information, it would have been important to gain a clear understanding of the patient's baseline, given his diagnosis of COPD. Patients with underlying airway disease often have chronic cough and some degree of shortness of breath. The presence of cough *or* shortness of breath means nothing in this population without comparing it to the patient's baseline.

## Timing and Duration

The emergency physician and the cardiovascular clinician elicited that the cough had been present for a month and the patient had sought treatment after 1 week. Both providers were also able to discover that his symptoms persisted to the point where he was exhausted, prompting his visit to the emergency department.

The cardiovascular clinician pursued one area of questioning that was overlooked by the emergency physician. Do you know what it was?

The emergency physician failed to ask about any activity that triggered the cough. The cardiovascular clinician asked this specifically—that is, whether the cough was triggered at certain times—and learned that the patient coughed more when lying flat. This positional worsening of his symptoms, in turn, caused him to sleep upright in a recliner and, in fact, the patient had been spending most of his day in this position due to loss of sleep and fatigue. He was also asked whether eating contributed to his cough. This is an important consideration, which we discuss a bit later.

## Associated Symptoms

The emergency physician asked about associated symptoms of fevers, shortness of breath, chest pain, dizziness, nausea or vomiting, or abnormal bleeding. The cardiovascular clinician was a bit more specific when asking about associated symptoms. We have learned that patients may experience chest discomfort that they do not consider to be pain, so it is important to differentiate between the two during the interview.

The cardiovascular provider also asked specifically about hemoptysis, which, when associated with cough, can raise concerns for malignancy in certain clinical contexts. The consulting cardiovascular clinician already knew there was objective evidence of heart failure on chest film. Atrial fibrillation can be both a trigger for and a result of heart failure exacerbations. In light of the patient's prior history, the clinician's line of questioning was also specific in seeking to determine whether he might be having breakthrough atrial fibrillation. Untreated sleep apnea can also trigger atrial fibrillation and increases in blood pressure. The patient was also questioned about CPAP compliance for this reason. In addition, the cardiovascular clinician asked specifically about weight changes, as well as swelling and dietary indiscretions that might have precipitated the heart failure.

When you are talking with a patient and obtaining a history, it is important to seek details not only about symptoms, but also about potential causes of those symptoms. You should always be thinking through your differential diagnosis list while simultaneously gathering the history and evaluating the patient.

## Mitigating or Alleviating Factors

Both providers asked the patient whether he took anything to alleviate his cough. He used his inhaler but had no relief. Both providers also learned that he had sought treatment elsewhere and had been treated for a COPD exacerbation; however, this treatment also did not relieve his symptoms.

The positional component of the cough is a factor that can also be quantified as a mitigating factor. Although the cough is present much of the time, lying down seems to precipitate it further, suggesting it is a trigger of sorts. It was not worsened with eating. In addition, both providers asked the patient about allergies, which can be an important component in patients who cough. No other factors seemed to mitigate or alleviate it.

# KEY FEATURES OF THE DATA

The key features of data in this case and with any complaint of cough are the laboratory data—looking for signs of infection—as well as the chest film. The vital signs, physical exam, and any relevant feature of the history continue to be important, as well. Let us discuss the data further.

## Vital Signs

Recall that the following findings were obtained by the cardiovascular clinician:

*Blood pressure:* Left arm, 166/80 mmHg; right arm, 172/82 mmHg

*Pulse:* approximately 70 beats per minute

*Respirations:* 16 breaths per minute

*Oxygen saturation:* 95% on room air

*Temperature:* 36.6°C

This patient was hypertensive on arrival to the emergency department. He noted his blood pressure had been elevated for the past few weeks. Uncontrolled hypertension can be a trigger in heart failure exacerbations. Perhaps this is a part of the problem.

## Electrocardiogram (ECG)

The ECG was reviewed by the cardiovascular clinician. It showed normal sinus rhythm. There were no abnormalities to suggest ischemia or any other underlying process. A repeat ECG did not show any changes.

## Chest Radiograph

The chest film in this case contained a crucial piece of information. It showed evidence of pulmonary edema and pleural effusions. This finding certainly explains the patient's persistent cough and is consistent with a picture of heart failure. Based on the chest film, we now know the "what," but we do not yet know the "why."

## Biomarkers and Lab Results

The only pertinent findings on the laboratory data were a WBC count in upper limits of normal, at 10,000, and a BNP level of 269 pg/mL. The marginal rise in his WBC count is not too concerning just yet, but it is worth repeating the test. Often such elevation results from a stress response or treatment with steroids. This patient was treated recently for a COPD exacerbation. If steroids were used, the WBC count might still be returning to normal levels a few weeks later. If the chest film was suspicious for an infectious process, the slightly elevated WBC count might be more worrisome, and further workup for an underlying infection might be pursued.

## Other Data

The patient's medical history was obtained throughout the evaluation. He was questioned specifically about the atrial fibrillation, sleep apnea, and the coronary artery disease, as these can be triggers of heart failure. In addition, he was asked about his blood pressure control and his baseline readings to further assess whether the current readings were deviations from the baseline.

His medications and compliance were confirmed. The list was as follows: warfarin, 2.5 mg daily; diltiazem XT (extended release), 120 mg daily; aspirin, 81 mg daily; atorvastatin, 80 mg at night; metformin, 1,000 mg twice daily before meals; fluticasone/salmeterol, 250 mcg/50 mcg daily; and a multivitamin daily. To evaluate whether management of his diabetes and high cholesterol is adequate, the patient's glycosylated hemoglobin and lipid panel should be checked every 3 months. The patient is questioned about this and reports that he was told his "numbers were good" at his last checkup 2 months ago. He confirms that he was placed on an antibiotic as well as a steroid dose pack for his COPD flare-up. Treatment finished a week ago.

His surgical history is significant for an inguinal hernia repair 3 years ago, cholecystectomy, and tonsillectomy. He is a former smoker, and no longer drinks. He does not use any illicit drugs. He is retired from the Navy and is widowed. He lives alone but has a daughter who helps take care of him and prepares his meals. His family history is unremarkable.

# DIFFERENTIALS AND DIFFERENCES IN EXAM

In a patient who presents with cough, the cardiorespiratory portion of the exam is the most important. Lung sounds, chest symmetry, expansion, and assessment of heart sounds can be the key to a diagnosis. We already know that the radiographic evidence supports heart failure in this patient, so what other pieces of the exam are important? The clinician should look carefully for jugular venous distension and edema, and also assess whether the patient is cool or warm.

The cardiovascular clinician examines the patient and notes these findings:

*General appearance: Well-nourished, morbidly obese White male in no acute distress.*

*Head and neck: Head is normocephalic and atraumatic, without evidence of lesions or masses. Sclera are anicteric. Neck is soft and supple, without thyromegaly or lymphadenopathy.*

*Cardiac exam: Assessment of jugular veins is difficult due to body habitus. There is elevation of jugular venous pressure to approximately 10 cm H2O. No carotid bruits. No femoral or abdominal bruits. Carotid upstrokes are symmetric and brisk. Peripheral pulses are palpable and symmetric. Auscultation of the heart reveals distant heart tones, a regular rate and rhythm, S1 and S2 present, soft S4. No murmurs or rubs. Chest wall is nontender to palpation.*

*Lungs: Diminished breath sounds bilaterally in bases with scattered crackles primarily in lower lobes bilaterally. Bilateral diffuse inspiratory and expiratory wheezing noted anteriorly. Symmetric expansion noted.*

*Abdomen:* Obese. Nontender. Bowel sounds present in all four quadrants. No hepatosplenomegaly. No hepatojugular reflux.

*Extremities:* Warm and dry. 2+ edema in bilateral ankles. 3 to 4+ massive scrotal edema noted with 4+ pitting edema in the sacrum and posterior thighs. No clubbing or cyanosis.

*Neurological:* Alert and oriented ×3. Cranial nerves are intact. Motor strength is symmetric in bilateral upper and lower extremities. No focal neurological deficits.

The patient has been thoroughly examined by both the emergency physician and the cardiovascular clinician. All key information has been obtained. We know from the objective data that this patient has heart failure, but we might have been led to that possibility through the history obtained by the cardiovascular clinician (history B), alone. History A, obtained in the emergency department, still led to the appropriate workup, but it did not necessarily direct suspicion to heart failure as the cause of the cough.

The exams performed by the two providers also differed, with the consulting clinician's examination leading to a more significant picture of volume overload than was initially presented. Although we have established a diagnosis, let us look more closely at some of the differential diagnoses of cough.

**Differential Diagnoses of Cough**

- Allergen/Pollution
- Disease (GERD)
- Gastroesophageal reflux
- Heart failure
- Infection
- Medication
- Postnasal drip
- Psychological
- Reactive airway disease

GERD, Gastroesophageal reflux disease.

# PUTTING IT ALL TOGETHER

## Working Through the Differential

Let us review these other causes of cough briefly and discuss why they might, or might not, be contributing to this clinical scenario.

Infection is always the first consideration when a patient presents with cough. This patient's cough had persisted for a month but he never had any fevers or other symptoms of infection. Although his WBC count is slightly elevated, it is unlikely to be due to infection. More likely this is a stress response or related to recent use of steroids, prescribed by his family physician to manage a suspected COPD exacerbation. Typically, when the WBC count is elevated from glucocorticoid use, the "left shift" seen with bacterial infections is absent; so, a CBC with differential can often aid in differentiating the two (Bushi, 2015). Aside from the WBC count, the chest film was also negative for any infectious process, so the cough is likely not due to infection.

We already know that this patient has COPD, which is a type of reactive airway disease. Heart failure and COPD have many overlapping features, making them difficult to distinguish in many cases. The two conditions can also coexist, increasing the challenge for clinicians in determining which process is causing the majority of a patient's symptoms. Heart failure is present in one in five patients with COPD exacerbations (Marcun et al., 2016).

The patient was very helpful in giving details about the baseline cough that he experiences with COPD. Chronic cough with and without sputum production is common among patients with underlying COPD. This patient was very clear that the cough causing him to seek treatment was different than his baseline cough. Unfortunately, it is common to assume that a new or worsening cough signifies a COPD exacerbation. He was treated for such an exacerbation by his family physician but did not improve. Although cough may be a component of his COPD, the positional nature and the concomitant exam findings point against COPD exacerbation as a *primary* cause of his cough at this time.

The cardiovascular clinician asked the patient whether there was any relationship between the cough and eating, and also asked if the patient had any symptoms of burning in his chest. These questions were specifically asked to determine whether GERD might be triggering his cough. GERD is a very common cause of chronic cough, and many of those affected require treatment for acid suppression (Houghton & Smith, 2017). A cough related to GERD may also occur more frequently when the individual is supine. However, in this case, GERD is unlikely to be the trigger for his cough based on the following:

- No symptoms of burning or history of heartburn
- No relationship to eating
- Cough has been present for only a month (i.e., chronicity has not been established)

We can also eliminate allergies, postnasal drip, and medication effect from the list of possible causes of this patient's cough for the following reasons:

- He has no allergies and has had no exposure to any new environmental triggers.
- He has no runny nose or symptoms of postnasal drip.
- He has been on the same medication without any changes that correlate with the timing of his cough.

This patient has clear evidence of a physical trigger for his cough; therefore, psychological causes can also be eliminated.

Let us talk about heart failure. There were key features about the patient's history and presentation suggestive of heart failure that the clinician was able to identify during the evaluation. Here are the high-lighted features from history B that should have supported the suspicion of heart failure:

- Cough noted when lying flat to sleep (orthopnea equivalent)
- Blood pressure elevated for the past few weeks
- Dietary indiscretion
- Predisposition with underlying obesity and hypertension

The physical exam findings further supported a diagnosis of heart failure. The patient denied any weight gain, although he admittedly did not weigh himself daily. He also denied any swelling. He was initially examined by the emergency physician and was found to have only mild lower extremity edema. Since the patient had not mentioned scrotal edema, this portion of the exam was likely deferred. There was something in the history that the consulting clinician discovered that prompted a deeper assessment for edema. Do you know what that was?

The patient had admitted to spending most of his day in the recliner. In an obese patient, the degree of edema is hard to ascertain, but the cardiovascular clinician suspected that perhaps he had more dependent edema in his sacrum, posterior legs, and even his scrotum due to his reduced activity and prolonged sitting position. Most patients might have mentioned the significant scrotal swelling, particularly when asked about swelling, but perhaps this patient did not see its relevance or was not bothered enough by it—or was embarrassed to mention it. It is important to look for dependent edema in these areas, particularly in this patient population. Although wheezing was present on the lung exam, this can be present in both heart failure and COPD.

In summary, the physical exam findings supporting a diagnosis of heart failure were as follows:

- Elevated jugular venous pressure
- Edema in sacrum, scrotum, legs
- Crackles and wheezing in lungs

The chest film showed evidence of pleural effusions and pulmonary edema, which was enough to explain the cough. A BNP level was also obtained, but showed only mild elevation. Many factors that can cause elevated BNP are not due to heart failure; additionally, there are many reasons this number can be lower than anticipated. It is important to understand that BNP levels increase with age but tend to be lower in obese patients, in the presence of lung disease, and in heart failure with preserved ejection fraction compared to heart failure with reduced ejection fraction (Januzzi & Mann, 2015). Hypertension is the most common cause of heart failure with preserved ejection fraction and is present in 85% of this population (Zile & Little, 2015). Obesity increases the risk of both heart failure and diastolic dysfunction.

Based on this patient's presentation, do you think he has heart failure with preserved or reduced ejection fraction? Can you tell just by physical exam?

The answer is no. Heart failure with preserved ejection fraction and reduced ejection fraction can have identical presentations. Only an echocardiogram can distinguish the two mechanisms with any certainty.

The patient's longstanding hypertension and obesity fit with the clinical picture of diastolic dysfunction, or heart failure with preserved ejection fraction, as confirmed by echocardiogram. However, to date he has not been diagnosed with heart failure. So, what do you think the "why" was?

The most likely precipitant was the increased salt intake in the patient's diet during his daughter's absence and the rise in blood pressure. These are common triggers for exacerbations in both heart failure with preserved ejection fraction and reduced ejection fraction. If the ejection fraction had been reduced, it would have been reasonable to evaluate for worsening coronary artery disease with coronary angiography.

**Likely Diagnosis**: Heart failure

---

WHAT'S NEXT?

- *This patient is admitted for new onset heart failure*
- An echocardiogram is performed that shows an ejection fraction of 59% and grade III diastolic dysfunction.
- The patient undergoes diuresis with intravenous furosemide over the course of 4 days and ultimately has a 20-pound reduction in weight with resolution of his cough. Daily diuretic therapy is added to his medication regimen.
- He is given education about heart failure, and the importance of medication, diet, and weight monitoring in management.

---

# SUMMARIZING THE SCENARIO

In most instances, a diagnosis of heart failure or a heart failure exacerbation can be made fairly quickly in the emergency department. This clinical scenario demonstrated how, in the right clinical context, a chief complaint of cough can and should be considered to reflect a heart failure symptom. Delayed diagnosis was averted because the chest film findings and elevated BNP raised concerns that led the emergency provider to request a cardiology consult. However, there was a clear difference in the history obtained by each provider, with history B supporting the suspicion of heart failure without the additional objective evidence.

The emergency physician may have thought the patient had a potentially mild heart failure exacerbation based on his lack of shortness of breath and mild physical exam findings. The cardiovascular clinician's clinical suspicion prompted a deeper examination for edema, which was more profound than initially suspected requiring hospitalization and intravenous diuresis.

The important highlights to take away from this case are:

- Edema can be difficult to assess in obese patients.
- Changes in weight and personal perception of swelling and weight gain may be altered in this population.
- Significant edema can hide in the sacrum, scrotum, and posterior thighs and these areas should always be examined, particularly if heart failure is suspected.
- Baseline presence of cough and shortness of breath should always be assessed in patients with COPD in order to establish changes.
- Nocturnal cough can be the equivalent of orthopnea.
- BNP values may not reflect the severity of volume overload in obese patients.

Experts in the field of cardiology are called upon to help identify sometimes subtle nuances of various disease processes. As always, the history is very important when assessing a complaint of cough as it can be indicative of multiple causes. When gathering information about the presentation, your goal is not only to try to identify every detail related to the chief complaint, but also to ask questions in a way that simultaneously excludes some differential diagnoses from your list.

# REFERENCES

Bushi, A. (2015). A general review of the mechanisms for steroid or glucocorticoid induced increases in the white blood cell count. Retrieved from http://www.ebmconsult.com/articles/steroids-glucocorticoids-wbc-neutrophiles-increse

Collins English Dictionary-Complete and Unabridged. (2014). Cough. Retrieved from http://www.thefreedictionary.com/cough

Houghton, L., & Smith, J. (2017). Gastro-oesophageal reflux events: Just another trigger in chronic cough? *Gut, 66*(12). doi:10.1136/gutjnl-2017-314027

Januzzi, J., & Mann, D. (2015). Clinical assessment of heart failure. In D. L. Mann, D. P. Zipes, P. Libby, & R. O. Bonow, *Braunwald's heart disease: A textbook of cardiovascular medicine* (10th ed., 473–483). Philadelphia, PA: Elsevier/Saunders.

Marcun, R., Stankovic, I., Vidakovic, R., Farkas, J., Kadivec, S., Putnikov, B., ... Lainscak, M. (2016). Prognostic implications of heart failure with preserved ejection fraction in patients with an exacerbation of chronic obstructive pulmonary disease. *Internal and Emergency Medicine, 11*(4), 519–527.

Rui, P., Kang, K., & Albert, M. (2013). National Hospital Medical Care Survey: 2013 emergency department summary tables. Retrieved from http://www.cdc.gov/nchs/data/ahcd/nhamcs_emergency/2013_ed_web_tables.pdf

Zile, M., & Little, W. (2015). Heart failure with preserved ejection fraction. In D. L. Mann, D. P. Zipes, P. Libby, R. O. Bonow, *Braunwald's heart disease: A textbook of cardiovascular medicine* (10th ed., pp. 557–574). Philadelphia, PA: Elsevier/Saunders.

# CHAPTER **11**

# Abdominal Pain

## DEFINITION AND CLINICAL SIGNIFICANCE OF ABDOMINAL PAIN

Abdominal pain is defined by *Segen's Medical Dictionary* (2011) as "a generic term for focal or general discomfort localized to the abdominal region." Abdominal pain is a common reason patients present in an acute care setting, representing around 10 million emergency department visits in 2013 according to the National Hospital Ambulatory Medical Care Survey (Rui, Kang, & Albert, 2013). The presence of abdominal pain can indicate any number of abnormalities, ranging from fairly benign and self-limiting to life threatening.

Other symptoms often accompany abdominal pain; these include nausea, vomiting, or changes in bowel patterns. But often it occurs in isolation. Patients frequently live with abdominal pain for several days to weeks before seeking medical attention. In other cases, the pain is so acute in onset and severity that immediate medical attention is required.

Initially patients may feel that pain in their abdomen indicates a problem in the abdominal cavity, but the abdomen is a common site for referred pain from other areas. Clinicians must be familiar with all the conditions that may manifest as abdominal pain and be hypervigilant in evaluating for the most acute among those possibilities.

As with other presentations, the history remains a critical piece in the evaluation of any patient with abdominal pain. It is important to determine whether the pain is acute or chronic, and to establish any and all factors that might be associated with it. As we have learned, patients may not give you, unprompted, all the information necessary to make an accurate diagnosis based on the history. Thorough and detailed questions are required to extract the information necessary to appropriately manage the symptoms.

Let us look at the following clinical scenario, reviewing the contrasting histories obtained by the providers who evaluate the patient.

## CASE SCENARIO

A 43-year-old African American male is brought to the emergency department by emergency medical services (EMS) with severe abdominal pain. He was at the gym when he experienced sudden abdominal pain with a sense of foreboding prompting him to ask others present to call 911. On arrival, he is diaphoretic and clammy. Blood pressure is 155/76 mmHg, pulse is 90 beats per minute, oxygen saturation is 98% on room air, and respirations are 18 breaths per minute. He is afebrile.

The emergency physician greets the patient and asks the following questions:

Q: **Can you tell me what happened?**

A: I was on the elliptical machine and I suddenly felt this excruciating, searing pain all along my abdomen. It's the worst pain of my life.

Q: **What did you do when you first felt it?**

A: I got down to the floor and doubled over. I thought I was going to pass out. I really felt like I was going to die—so I yelled for help.

Q: **How do you feel now?**

A: Horrible. Something is really wrong.

Q: **Did you have or are you having any chest pain, nausea, vomiting, or shortness of breath?**

A: I'm a little nauseated, but nothing else.

Q: **Can you describe the pain for me? Is it sharp, stabbing, throbbing, squeezing?**

   A: It feels like someone is stabbing me from the inside out, but squeezing my sides at the same time.

Q: **Is the pain in one particular spot on your abdomen or is it all over?**

   A: I feel it everywhere—from my ribs to below my shorts.

Q: **How long were you working out before this happened?**

   A: I had just gotten to the gym about 25 minutes before. I finished lifting weights and was starting my cardio routine.

Q: **Did you have any pain when you were lifting weights or did you feel anything out of the ordinary?**

   A: No. I felt fine.

Q: **Have you been sick recently or felt unwell leading up to today, or had anything different in your diet?**

   A: Not at all.

Q: **Do you have any history of heart attack, stroke, or abdominal issues?**

   A: No. I have high blood pressure and I take medication for it. But that's it.

Q: **Have you noticed any bleeding in your stool or urine?**

   A: No.

At this point the emergency physician notes that the patient is becoming restless with obvious distress. He is quickly examined, and the data are obtained and reviewed. The exam is unremarkable for any significant findings. Guarding of the abdomen is noted; however, the abdomen is only mildly tender to palpation. An ECG is obtained and shows deep T-wave inversion in the inferior leads. Sublingual nitroglycerin is given without any significant change in the patient's pain. Laboratory data are ordered, and results are pending. The chest film did not show any abnormalities. Because of the ECG findings and the concern for possible myocardial ischemia, a cardiology consult is requested for urgent evaluation.

The emergency physician relays the following information to the cardiovascular clinician:

## History A

*A 43-year-old African American male with a past medical history of hypertension who was in his usual state of health was brought to the emergency department by EMS with complaints of severe abdominal pain. The pain started abruptly while the patient was at the gym after lifting weights and was associated with diaphoresis, nausea, near syncope, and a sense of doom. He denies any associated chest pain, vomiting, or shortness of breath. He denies any recent illness, change in his diet, or bleeding. Blood pressure and pulse were mildly elevated on arrival. Chest film is normal; however, ECG shows significant T-wave inversion in the inferior leads. Laboratory data are pending, but there is concern for an acute coronary syndrome (ACS); therefore, we need cardiology assistance for management.*

The consulting cardiology clinician quickly arrives to evaluate the patient. Repeat vital signs are obtained, as follows:

*Blood pressure*: Right arm, 130/65 mmHg; left arm, 146/80 mmHg

*Pulse*: 82 beats per minute

*Respirations*: 16 breaths per minute

*Oxygen saturation*: 97% on room air

*Temperature*: 37.0°C

A repeat ECG is also obtained that shows worsening T-wave inversion in the inferior leads.

The cardiovascular clinician asks the patient the following questions:

Q: **I know you are uncomfortable, but can you tell me what happened today?**

A: I was working out at the gym and I had this sudden, severe pain in my abdomen. I've never felt anything like it.

Q: **What did you do when you felt it?**

A: I got down to the floor and doubled over. I yelled for help.

Q: **Can you describe it for me? Is it stabbing, sharp, tearing, squeezing, throbbing, dull, or something else?**

A: It feels like there is a stabbing from my insides, but then it also feels like there is a vice pushing on me from the outside. It's searing.

Q: **Can you point to where it hurts?**

A: All over (he proceeds to point from his epigastric region to his pelvis).

Q: **Are you having any chest pain, back pain, jaw pain, or arm pain?**

A: No.

Q: **Are you having any shortness of breath, nausea, vomiting, or dizziness?**

A: I am a little nauseated. I thought I was going to pass out from the pain but I didn't.

Q: **What were you doing, exactly, when it occurred?**

A: I had just gotten on the elliptical, didn't even really start, and I felt it and dropped to the floor. I yelled for help—I thought I was going to die.

Q: **I understand you were lifting weights just before that. Did you lift more than usual or have any discomfort during it?**

A: No. I have the same routine and it felt fine.

Q: **Have you been sick recently? Any fevers or sick contacts?**

A: No.

Q: **Any diarrhea, constipation, or blood in your stool? Any problems urinating or blood in your urine?**

A: No. I had a bowel movement last night and it was normal. I felt fine until this happened. I don't have any trouble urinating.

Q: **I see you have a history of high blood pressure. Do you have any history of high cholesterol, heart disease, diabetes, or thyroid problems?**

A: No, just high blood pressure.

Q: **Have you ever been told you have any heart problems or valve problems? Ever had a heart catheterization or stress test?**

A: No.

Q: **Have you ever had a stroke, heart attack, or blood clot in your lungs or legs?**

A: No.

Q: **Have you ever had any problems with your digestive system? Have you ever been diagnosed with an abdominal problem?**

A: No.

Q: **Do you have any history of cancer, or any surgeries or injuries?**

A: No cancer. I hurt my knee playing college basketball once, but nothing else.

Q: **Have you been in any accidents or had any falls recently?**

A: No.

Q: **Are you having any numbness or tingling in your legs or arms?**

A: No, I don't think so. My feet feel cold, but I don't think that's anything.

Q: **When this pain came on, did you feel any ripping or tearing, or hear any popping sounds?**

A: Now that you mention it, I felt a pop—deep inside I think.

Q: **Are you on any blood-thinning medication?**

A: No.

Q: **Do you smoke or drink? Do you use any drugs?**

A: I drink occasionally. I've never smoked or done any drugs.

Q: **Any family history of heart attacks, heart disease, or stroke?**

A: My dad died at 38 of a massive heart attack. My mom has high blood pressure, like me.

The cardiovascular clinician completes a physical exam and reviews the laboratory data; we discuss those findings a bit later. The clinician's history of present illness is summarized as follows:

## History B

*A 43-year-old African American male with a history only of hypertension was brought to the emergency department by EMS with complaints of abrupt onset* of severe abdominal pain while at the gym associated with a sense of doom. He had been in his usual state of health and had just completed his normal weight-lifting routine when he proceeded to step onto the elliptical and suddenly experienced the discomfort. He describes it as a stabbing, searing, yet vicelike pain radiating throughout his abdomen from his epigastric region to his pelvis. He recalls feeling a "popping" sensation just before the pain came on. He denies any chest pain, back pain, arm pain, or shortness of breath. He is diaphoretic with nausea and had near syncope initially, but denies any vomiting. He denies any numbness or tingling in the extremities but reports that his feet feel cold. He denies any changes to his diet or bowel pattern and denies any melena, hematochezia, or hematuria.

He has had no recent accidents or illnesses. He has no cardiovascular history or history of abdominal conditions. He does not take any blood-thinning medication. He has a history of premature coronary artery disease in his family. His father died of a massive heart attack at the age of 38. He denies any illicit drug use or tobacco use, but does drink occasionally. He has never experienced anything like this prior to today. His ECG raised concerns for a possible ACS, and he was treated with nitroglycerin without any major change in his symptoms.

Based on this history, do you have any differential diagnoses in mind other than an ACS? What should your immediate next step be? Let us dive deeper.

## KEY FEATURES OF THE HISTORY

When patients present to the emergency department via EMS, often an acute situation *becomes* one of urgency. Many times, these patients are unstable, or so uncomfortable that taking a history becomes limited by time and the severity of the situation. It is still important to gather as much information as possible in order to formulate the most likely diagnosis and the best management plan. In these cases, the cardiovascular clinician is often the third person to evaluate the patient, after paramedics and the emergency physician. Information is often shared among these providers in order to populate an accurate picture of what has happened when the patient may not be able to continue to provide information.

In clinical situations of urgency, the history is often taken simultaneously while the patient is being examined, while ECGs are obtained, and while laboratory tests are gathered. Often, as here, all the data may not be available at the time you are asked to evaluate the patient. Therefore, you become reliant on your history and physical exam to direct the next steps in the workup of the patient.

In a clinical presentation of abdominal pain, it is important to determine the nature, onset, and timing of the pain; any associated factors; and any factors that may have precipitated it. Once these are defined, the broad differential of abdominal pain can be narrowed significantly, making a diagnosis much easier to determine.

Let us review the key features of the history in this case.

## Character

Each provider assessed the character of this patient's abdominal pain and learned that it was severe, stabbing, searing, and vicelike. In addition, the pain did not localize to one specific region of the abdomen, but rather extended from the epigastric region to the pelvis. In the setting of abdominal pain these descriptive characteristics are monumental clues in determining the cause. Each history demonstrated these features adequately.

## Timing and Duration

Both the emergency physician and the cardiovascular clinician learned that the pain was abrupt in onset and has continued since it began. The patient disclosed that this was "the worst pain of his life," and that he has never experienced anything like it. Abdominal pain that is sudden in onset does not typically have the same cause as abdominal pain that is more gradual in onset. This feature portends a more acute and potentially life-threatening condition. It should certainly relay a sense of urgency in determining the diagnosis.

## Associated Symptoms

The emergency physician asked the patient whether he was feeling any associated symptoms, such as chest pain, nausea, vomiting, or shortness of breath, and also asked about any recent illness or bleeding issues. The cardiovascular clinician asked about the same issues, but expanded the questions to include jaw pain, arm pain, fever, bowel patterns, dizziness, and numbness or tingling in the extremities. The patient revealed to both providers that he was nauseated and felt as if he was going to pass out initially from the pain. He had diaphoresis on presentation and revealed that he had an associated sense of doom. Although he did not have any neurological symptoms, he did mention—in response to prompting—that his feet were cold.

In addition to eliciting more comprehensive assessment of the associated symptoms, the cardiovascular clinician asked if the patient had felt or heard any popping or tearing sounds at the time his pain began. He did not mention this, unprompted, to the first provider or to the EMS personnel, but he responded to the consulting clinician's direct question by stating that he did, in fact, feel a deep "pop" inside. This detail turns out to be one of the most critical pieces of information, as we discuss a bit later, and further reinforces a point made in earlier chapters—that often patients do not remember these types of details, do not think they are relevant, or are simply too uncomfortable to mention them on their own without being asked directly.

Do you think anything in particular prompted the cardiovascular clinician to ask this question?

## Mitigating or Alleviating Factors

Both clinicians identified that the patient was at the gym just before the onset of pain. He was asked whether he felt poorly at any time prior to the event and during his weightlifting. In attempting to define a potential trigger, the cardiovascular clinician asked the patient if he had changed his weightlifting routine to one that was harder than usual. He was also asked specifically about any recent accidents or injuries, which can often precipitate abdominal injury. Again, this questioning was pursued to determine whether trauma was in any way a mitigating factor.

The patient's pain was sudden in onset, and he did not have much time prior to the arrival of EMS personnel to alleviate the pain himself. He did tell both providers that he got down on the floor quickly, doubled over, and called for help. Despite these actions, the severity of the pain did not improve. Once the ECG was obtained, he was given nitroglycerin, which did not alleviate his symptoms to any significant degree. So, no clear mitigating or alleviating factors have been defined.

# KEY FEATURES OF THE DATA

As previously noted, only a few key features of the data were available at the time the cardiovascular clinician evaluated the patient. The clinician had already established a working diagnosis based on the history, limited data, and physical exam. The completion of the laboratory data only supplemented the initial suspicion. Let us review the data further.

## Vital Signs

Vital signs assess for hemodynamic stability in acute presentations. The blood pressure obtained by the paramedics at the scene was 155/76 mm/Hg. The patient's heart rate was slightly elevated, at 90 beats per minute, and the oxygen saturation as well as respiratory rate were reasonable. When the clinician first came to evaluate the patient, the vital signs were repeated and blood pressures were taken in both arms. Remember, at this point, the patient had already received a sublingual nitroglycerin tablet. The following findings were reported:

*Blood pressure:* Right arm, 130/65 mmHg; left arm, 146/80 mmHg

*Pulse:* 82 beats per minute

*Respirations:* 16 breaths per minute

*Oxygen saturation:* 97% on room air

*Temperature:* 37.0°C

Do you notice any abnormality? It is essential to make it part of your practice to check blood pressures in *each* arm in order to assess for any degree of difference. In this scenario, this finding makes a critical difference in the next management steps for this patient, as we discuss shortly.

## Electrocardiogram (ECG)

The abnormality noted on the ECG was the trigger to involve the cardiovascular clinician in this case. The ECG demonstrated normal sinus rhythm with normal QRS duration but deep T-wave inversions that worsened on repeat ECG, prompting consideration of an ACS workup. These findings certainly raise concern for ischemia, but what else could they mean?

## Chest Radiograph

The chest film showed no evidence of pulmonary disease, edema, or infection. There was no cardiomegaly, and the mediastinum was not widened.

## Biomarkers and Lab Results

The laboratory data were reviewed. The CBC was within normal limits, and the chemistry panel showed no significant abnormalities. Liver function studies were normal, as were amylase and lipase levels. The troponin T level was 0.04 ng/mL and the D-dimer was 8.2 mcg/mL fibrinogen equivalent units (FEU). These abnormal values should enable you to narrow your differential even further.

## Other Data

During the course of the evaluation, the patient's medication list was reviewed. He takes lisinopril, 20 mg daily, as well as hydrochlorothiazide (HCTZ), 12.5 mg daily, for his hypertension. He admits to compliance. Thorough questioning reveals no other pertinent medical history. His surgical history is negative. He has a positive family history for premature coronary artery disease in his father and hypertension in his mother. He admitted to occasional alcohol use but no tobacco or other drugs. He is active and otherwise healthy and exercises on a regular basis.

# DIFFERENTIALS AND DIFFERENCES IN EXAM

Aside from the history, the physical exam remains the second most critical part of evaluating any patient—particularly in an urgent situation. Careful, quick, yet thorough examination is required to help support or dismiss any potential working diagnosis.

The cardiovascular clinician's findings on examination of the patient are as follows:

*General appearance:* Well-nourished, physically fit African American male in a moderate amount of distress.

*Head and neck:* Head is normocephalic and atraumatic, without evidence of lesions or masses. Sclera are anicteric. Neck is soft and supple, without thyromegaly or lymphadenopathy.

*Cardiac exam:* There is no elevation of jugular venous pressure. No carotid bruits. No femoral or abdominal bruits. Carotid upstrokes are symmetric and brisk. Peripheral pulses are palpable but asymmetric, with reduced strength in right arm and in bilateral lower extremities. Auscultation of the heart reveals a regular rate and rhythm, S1 and S2 present. No S3 or S4. No murmurs or rubs. Chest wall is nontender to palpation.

*Lungs:* Clear lung sounds in bilateral lung fields. Symmetric expansion noted.

*Abdomen:* Soft, but guarded, slightly tender to deep palpation. Bowel sounds present in all four quadrants. No hepatosplenomegaly. No hepatojugular reflux.

*Extremities:* Diaphoretic and clammy, but warm. Bilateral lower extremities are slightly colder to palpation. No clubbing or cyanosis.

*Neurological:* Alert and oriented ×3. Cranial nerves are intact. Motor strength is symmetric in bilateral upper and lower extremities. Sensation is intact. No focal neurological deficits.

At this point all key information has been gathered. Based on what you know now, do you think this is a presentation of ACS?

Both history A and history B identified important features of the clinical presentation. The cardiovascular clinician identified a few other critical pieces of information that should lead you to focus on ruling in or ruling out only one diagnosis at this point. The abrupt onset of the pain, its severity, and the associated "popping" sensation and pulse deficits should lead you to acute aortic dissection as the most likely diagnosis. This working diagnosis must rapidly be confirmed by contrast CT scan or death could be imminent.

For the sake of discussion, however, let us look at other differential diagnoses for acute abdominal pain that might also be considered in this clinical scenario.

Differential Diagnoses of Abdominal Pain

- Acute cholecystitis
- Acute pancreatitis
- ACS
- Aortic dissection
- Appendicitis
- Cholangitis
- Colitis

- Gastroenteritis
- Hernia
- Mass
- Mesenteric ischemia
- Nephrolithiasis
- Peptic ulcer
- Peritonitis

- Pulmonary embolus
- Ruptured abdominal aortic aneurysm
- Small bowel obstruction
- Testicular torsion

ACS, acute coronary syndrome.

This list certainly does not cover all the potential causes for abdominal pain, but these are some of the diagnoses you should have in mind when evaluating any patient with an acute abdomen.

# PULLING IT ALL TOGETHER

## Working Through the Differential

Cardiovascular clinicians do not routinely see patients and evaluate them for abdominal pain, so if we are involved it is usually because an abnormal cardiac finding in this setting prompts consideration of the abdominal pain as an atypical manifestation of a cardiac issue. Many of the conditions on the differentials list share common features, and it might be difficult to distinguish one from another at first. It is important to realize, however, that the presence of findings that are *most consistent* with one diagnosis is reason enough to rule out many of the others on the list.

In the opening scenario, the high degree of likelihood that this patient has an acute aortic dissection negates consideration of almost all the other differentials unless it is ruled out. These are merely other diagnoses that should be considered in most presentations of an acute abdominal pain. Additionally, many of these conditions are confirmed or ruled out with the same imaging tests. That being said, let us review only the diagnoses that fall into the cardiovascular category.

The patient's D-dimer is elevated. Could his abdominal pain represent a pulmonary embolus? Not likely—let us look at why.

- He is not short of breath.
- He is not tachycardic.
- Oxygenation is normal on room air.
- He has no risk factors for pulmonary embolus.

What about mesenteric ischemia? Depending on the mechanism of the ischemia, this often has a slower onset with more symptoms of nausea, diarrhea, and sometimes gastrointestinal bleeding. Underlying coronary artery disease, peripheral artery disease, and cerebrovascular disease are risk factors for mesenteric arterial thrombosis, which is one mechanism for mesenteric ischemia (Dang, 2016). Again, this presentation is gradual in onset, with pain that often occurs after eating. Mesenteric arterial embolization can have an acute onset with severe pain and vomiting with diarrhea. The mechanism is usually of cardiac origin, so these patients may have underlying atrial fibrillation or recent myocardial infarction (Dang, 2016).

Mesenteric ischemia can occur as a complication of acute aortic dissection and can also coincide with limb ischemia in patients with these symptoms (Charlton-Ouw et al., 2016). Usually the diagnosis of mesenteric ischemia is based on clinical suspicion in the presence of severe abdominal pain and confirmed with a CT scan. We can presume that primary mesenteric ischemia is not the cause of this patient's symptoms, but it should be considered in this case as a possible consequence of the acute aortic dissection. The urgent CT scan should include the chest and abdomen to confirm or rule out this suspicion.

Acute rupture of an abdominal aortic aneurysm can present very similarly to an aortic dissection, but there are a few differences. Gawenda and Brunkwall (2012) describe the classic triad of a ruptured aortic aneurysm:

- Pain in the abdomen and or back
- Hypotension
- Pulsatile abdominal mass

This patient demonstrates only one of these criteria, making acute ruptured abdominal aortic aneurysm less likely as a primary diagnosis.

Acute aortic dissection can mimic an ACS in many cases. It is very common for patients with an acute aortic dissection to present with ECG changes as well as elevated troponin levels. In fact, normal ECG findings in this population are rare (Pourafkari et al., 2016). The classic presentation of aortic dissection is chest pain and sometimes back pain, and patients with an ACS often present with abdominal pain as an atypical symptom or angina equivalent, which can make it much more challenging to distinguish between the two.

The most common ECG finding in acute aortic dissection is not necessarily ST elevation, but rather T-wave inversion (Pourafkari et al., 2016). The presence of coronary ischemia is a result of the dissection and leads to coronary malperfusion, typically in the right coronary artery distribution, which manifests in the inferior leads on ECG. This process is also evident in the elevated troponin levels. *Misdiagnosis can be fatal.* If an ACS is suspected, patients may be initiated on guideline-directed therapy with anticoagulants and IIb/IIA inhibitors, which can have catastrophic outcomes (Lentini & Perrotta, 2011). Whenever there is any clinical suspicion of an acute aortic dissection, urgent imaging needs to be done *prior to* the administration of therapy for ACS.

Acute aortic dissection is an uncommon condition with a very high mortality rate in which death often occurs prior to diagnosis and treatment. There are two types of aortic dissection, and two classifications are used, as detailed by Braverman (2015):

## DeBakey

- *Type I*: Ascending aorta; extends at least to the aortic arch and often to the descending aorta and beyond
- *Type II*: Confined to the ascending aorta, only
- *Type III*: Descending aorta; distal to the left subclavian artery extending distally

## Stanford

- *Type A*: Involving the ascending aorta with or without extension to the descending aorta
- *Type B*: Dissections not involving the ascending aorta

The classic presentation of patients with an aortic dissection is severe chest pain that may radiate through to the back and is often accompanied by a sense of doom. Often these patients describe the pain as a tearing sensation, or they may feel or hear a tearing or popping sound. Although rare, some patients have no symptoms of acute heart failure from the consequence of severe aortic regurgitation, syncope, or abdominal pain. Atypical presentations lead to misdiagnosis and often a higher mortality rate.

There is a higher incidence of aortic dissection among men aged 50 to 60 years, and hypertension is present in 70% of patients with acute aortic dissection (Braverman, 2015). Other underlying risk factors include congenital diseases of the aorta (e.g., Marfan's syndrome), drug use, bicuspid aortic valve, atherosclerosis, and trauma. Congenital abnormalities are more commonly present in younger patients. Clinical symptoms often mimic those of many other conditions, as we have demonstrated. The exam can be normal, there may be subtle findings, or patients can present in cardiac arrest or shock.

Exam findings that should trigger your clinical suspicion of aortic dissection in presentations such as this are:

- Presence of pulse deficits
- A murmur consistent with aortic regurgitation
- Neurological deficits

In addition to abnormal ECG findings and elevated troponin levels in aortic dissection, the D-dimer level can be elevated. The chest film may show a widened mediastinum or abnormal aortic arch contour, but not always. These findings are not specific for the diagnosis of aortic dissection, but in the right clinical context their presence should prompt further evaluation with imaging.

Let us review the findings in this case to demonstrate why aortic dissection was the most likely cause.

- Severe, abrupt abdominal pain associated with the feeling of "popping"
- Discrepancy in blood pressures
- Risk factor of being male and hypertensive

- Elevated D-dimer
- T-wave inversion on inferior leads
- Reduced temperature in lower extremities

Although these findings were subtle and can overlap with other conditions, even the slightest clinical suspicion of aortic dissection needs to be pursued because of the dire consequences otherwise.

**Likely Diagnosis:** Aortic dissection

---

## WHAT'S NEXT?

- *A contrast CT of the chest, abdomen, and pelvis with dissection protocol is ordered. The patient is found to have a Stanford type A dissection extending just proximally to the iliac arteries.*
- He is then taken for emergent surgical repair. No congenital abnormalities of the aorta or the aortic valve are noted.
- The patient makes a full recovery with no resultant deficits.

---

## SUMMARIZING THE SCENARIO

When cardiac clinicians think of acute aortic dissection, symptoms of chest pain, back pain, and stabbing and tearing qualities are foremost in our minds. We assume a widened mediastinum or variations in blood pressures will be present. These are the findings we look for most often when patients present with symptoms suggestive of dissection.

In medicine, however, we must always consider the atypical, the unusual, and the rare presentations—otherwise the outcome could be deadly. This case is a clear example of that rare and unusual circumstance. Cardiovascular clinicians do not often become involved when patients present with acute abdominal pain. The abnormal ECG triggered the consult and also the consideration that the pain might represent something outside the abdominal cavity.

This case, more so than others we have discussed in this book, highlights the need to always measure blood pressure in both arms. This small, yet significant, detail prompted specific questioning from the consulting clinician that not only supported the diagnosis, but also shifted the initial focus from treatment of ACS to evaluation for acute aortic dissection. If this patient had been started on anticoagulation or any therapies standard for ACS, the result would likely have been death.

This is not to say that imaging of the abdomen would not have been pursued otherwise. If we assume that the discrepancy in blood pressure had not been identified, in the absence of ST elevation on ECG it is plausible that dedicated CT of the abdomen would have been ordered. There might not have been urgent imaging of the chest with dissection protocol, however, and diagnosis might have been delayed. In acute aortic dissection, there is little time to waiver on diagnosis and management because the mortality rate is so high.

Aside from the pulse deficits, this patient had severe, abrupt pain that was later determined to be associated with a feeling of a "popping" sensation. That, accompanied by a sense of foreboding and feelings of death, signals the urgency of the situation. Although this patient was younger that most with dissection, he had two identified risk factors in being male and having chronic hypertension. Chronic hypertension is the most common risk factor for acute aortic dissection (Lee, Jourabchi, Sauk, & Lanum, 2013). Very few conditions that are not life-threatening are associated with a patient who reports a sense of doom. These are bold statements when made by the patient and necessitate rapid evaluation.

As clinicians, we must always be vigilant and think outside the box. Regardless of the specialty, it is important to consider which conditions can present atypically and what we should look for during the evaluation. The emergency physician demonstrated this vigilance when considering a possible ACS presenting as abdominal pain. This prompted appropriate involvement of the cardiovascular clinician, and the combined rapid assessment and treatment led to a positive outcome rather than a devastating one.

# REFERENCES

Braverman, A. (2015). Diseases of the aorta. In D. L. Mann, D. P. Zipes, P. Libby, & R. O. Bonow, *Braunwald's heart disease: A textbook of cardiovascular medicine* (10th ed., 1277–1311). Philadelphia, PA: Elsevier/Saunders.

Charlton-Ouw, K., Sandhu, H., Leake, S., Jeffress, K., Miller III., C., Durham, C., … Azizzadeh, A. (2016). Need for limb revascularization in patients with acute aortic dissection is associated with mesenteric ischemia. *Annals of Vascular Surgery, 36*, 112–120. doi:10.1016/.j.avsg.2016.03.012.

Dang, C. (2016). Acute mesenteric ischemia clinical presentation. Retrieved from http://www.emedicine.medscape.com/article/189146-clinical

Gawenda, M., & Brunkwall, J. (2012). Ruptured abdominal aortic aneurysm. *Deutsches Ärzteblatt International, 109*(43), 727–732. doi:10.3238/arztbl.2012.0727

Lee, E., Jourabchi, N., Sauk, S., & Lanum, D. (2013). An extensive Stanford type A aortic dissection involving bilateral carotid and iliac arteries. *Case Reports in Radiology, 2013.* doi:10.1155/2013/607012.

Lentini, S., & Perrota, S. (2011). Aortic dissection with concomitant acute myocardial infarction: From diagnosis to management. *Journal of Emergencies, Trauma, and Shock, 4*(2), 273–278. doi:10.4103/0974-2700.82221

Pourafkari, L., Tajlil, A., Ghaffari, S., Chavoshi, M., Kolahdouzan, K., Parvizi, R., … Parizad, R. (2016). Electrocardiography changes in acute aortic dissection-association with troponin leak, coronary anatomy and prognosis. *The American Journal of Emergency Medicine, 34*(8), 1431–1436.

Rui, P., Kang, K., & Albert, M. (2013). National Hospital Medical Care Survey: 2013 emergency department summary tables. Retrieved from http://www.cdc.gov/nchs/data/ahcd/nhamcs_emergency/2013_ed_web_tables.pdf

Segen's Medical Dictionary. (2011). Abdominal pain. Retrieved from http://medical-dictionary.thefreedictionary.com/abdominal+pain

# PART III

# Summary and Useful Clinical Tools

In this book, we discuss the importance of taking a comprehensive history when evaluating the patient with a suspected cardiac condition. Optimal treatment depends on obtaining key features of the history and putting it all together with the objective evidence to determine a potential diagnosis. Early in every provider's career, the process of obtaining these details is often fragmented, but as experience is gained—regardless of the specialty—providers learn to streamline their questioning to ensure a complete, pertinent—and timely—evaluation.

One of the most challenging parts of being a clinician is putting all of this information together and documenting it in a way that tells the patient's story, summarizing everything that needs to be portrayed—for the patient record and the next provider. In this book the workup format was broken down purposefully to delineate key elements of the history and other data. In Chapter 13, four scenarios that were presented in earlier chapters are written up to demonstrate how to structure the information into a standard (real-world) format as a way to tell the story and paint the picture.

# CHAPTER **12**

# Conclusion

In this book, we looked closely at both common and uncommon chief complaints of cardiac conditions and how differences in taking the history can lead the clinician in different directions. In the case scenarios provided, the history obtained by the emergency department provider was compared with that of the cardiovascular clinician who was called in to consult on the case. The intent was not to portray inadequacies in the initial provider's evaluation, but rather to demonstrate how the expertise of the cardiovascular clinician was called upon in determining whether an underlying cardiac condition existed when one might have been suspected. The approach was also used to demonstrate *which* cardiac condition was present when frequently a different one was suspected.

Taking a comprehensive history requires experience, expertise, and an extensive knowledge of various disease processes. The goal of the emergency department provider is to evaluate a patient in a timely fashion and determine the best course of action, which is often to consult a specialist, depending on the suspected diagnosis. It is the role of that specialist to dig deeper and acquire as much information as possible about the chief complaint in order to formulate the best management plan for the patient.

All healthcare providers learned the basics of taking a history during our training programs. It is not until we are exposed to various conditions and disease processes particular to our field of practice that we learn to fine-tune that skill and apply the knowledge we have gained to more specifically identify the ongoing problem. The goal of this book is to assimilate years of that exposure and experience in a format that will enable you to take a history with the skill and detail that is not typically acquired without those years of practice.

Throughout this book we have focused on key features of the chief complaint and dissected each one to demonstrate gaps in what might have been perceived, initially, to be a thorough history. Those key features were character (which includes location and severity), timing and duration, associated symptoms, and mitigating or alleviating factors. It is important to keep these features in mind when evaluating a patient with any chief complaint. To understand the complaint and determine a cause, you must ask everything you can about the symptom(s) and assume that patients will not tell you all the pertinent details unless they are asked.

For example, as cardiovascular clinicians we use the term "chest pain" to encompass any discomfort or sensation in the chest. However, as Chapters 3 and 4 demonstrated, many patients may not perceive their chest symptoms as pain, but instead as a pressure or a discomfort. Thus, if they are asked about chest pain, they may give a false negative answer. This example, and others throughout the book, prove how important it is to be very specific when assessing symptoms. Do not ask if patients have pain but rather if they have discomfort, pressure, pain, or any chest symptoms. *The more descriptive we are in our questioning, the more descriptive patients will be in their answers.*

Electronic medical records provide clinicians with access to the medication history and various other details of the history if a patient has been seen previously at that institution. As earlier chapters emphasize, clinicians must review that information specifically to assess for changes, rather than making assumptions about what is documented and whether it is still valid. Using information already contained in the medical record allows for a more timely evaluation, but important clues can be overlooked when clinicians do not take the time to review these details each time the patient presents. The electronic medical record should serve to guide our questions and be reviewed for pertinent background information, but it is not a substitute for a thorough and comprehensive assessment of the patient's history.

Patients are sometimes admitted and undergo expensive and exhaustive evaluations in order to confirm or disprove the presence of a critical underlying issue. This process is largely driven by medicolegal fears that may, at times, override clinical suspicion. Patients may not require costly tests, but clinicians who do not arrange for these tests may worry that something might be missed.

This book demonstrates that a diagnosis can often be made on the basis of a detailed and comprehensive history alone. In addition, by reviewing supportive exam findings and objective evidence, providers may determine that treatment does not require either admission or the imaging that might initially have been planned for a patient.

As the healthcare environment has changed, clinicians have been faced with a higher volume of patients who must be seen and less time in which to see them. Some might argue that there is not enough time to take a detailed history, and that it is easier and safer to opt for expensive testing. But learning as much as you can about the chief complaint is a benefit, leading to faster and more accurate diagnosis, treatment, and relief of symptoms for the patient. Also, spending more time evaluating the patient by means of a comprehensive exam and history on the front end may save the patient money on the back end.

Sometimes, abnormal lab values or tests can cause providers to narrow their focus and miss the bigger picture. Cardiovascular clinicians are often asked to evaluate patients for abnormal troponin levels or abnormal electrocardiographic findings. It is important to remember that these are only pieces of a larger pie. We must not become so sidetracked by abnormal findings that we fail to take a closer look at the clinical context in which they occur. *Remember, you are treating a patient, not a lab value.* Always look at the whole picture and consider all the possibilities for these findings in a particular clinical setting so the right diagnosis is not missed.

In the field of cardiology there are instances in which we do not have the luxury of time or patient stability to obtain all the information we want about the presenting symptom. Sometimes patients are too unstable or unable to give us any details because they are in distress. In these cases, we focus our evaluation on key questions while simultaneously performing an exam or obtaining lab data. Often a group effort by the paramedic team, emergency department provider, perhaps family members, and the cardiovascular clinician is required to exchange information and fill in the gaps in the history when the patient is unable to do so.

Many symptoms, both common and uncommon, can represent acute cardiac conditions. It is my hope that this book demonstrated not only the nuances of these conditions, but also key features to consider when taking a history and performing an exam in order to pinpoint the diagnosis when others might not be able to do so. Healthcare providers are investigators of sorts. Each piece of information we elicit is a clue. Everything we see, everything that is said, and even things that are unsaid are important. Always remember that there is no such thing as too many questions in medicine. What you will find out with an inquisitive mind is limitless. I hope this book proves that point.

In the Introduction, I stated that taking a history is an art, like painting a picture. You want that picture to be detailed, vivid, colorful, and full of dimension. Once that picture is painted, you want to be able to describe it in a way that enables someone who is not physically present to visualize it in exactly the same way as someone who is standing in front of it. That is what your documented history of present illness should look like—a beautifully crafted, skilled piece of art that rivals the work of the most experienced artists: a masterpiece. It is my hope that this book provided you with the skills to create masterpieces.

# Bonus Section: The Write-Up

This book discusses how to obtain a comprehensive history, identify key features of the patient evaluation, and determine a diagnosis. The elements of the history and evaluation are reviewed in Chapters 1 through 11. In this bonus chapter, the history and physical exam (H&P) for four of the cases presented earlier in the book are written up using a format similar to the standard patient chart to demonstrate how to put it all together. Chapter cross-references to each case scenario are listed for reference.

## SAMPLE WRITE-UP 1: H&P (Chapter 1 Case Scenario)

*Chief Complaint*
Chest pain and "burning"

*History of Present Illness (HPI)*
A 69-year-old (y/o) African American (AA) male with multiple cardio-vascular risk factors including known coronary artery disease (CAD) with prior stenting 4 years ago presents to the emergency department at 1900 with complaints of chest pain and burning. He describes the pain as more of a mild ache with a burning quality that is epigastric in nature. He noticed it about 11 a.m. while lying down after he just finished a late breakfast. He denies any acid brash associated with the pain. The pain was nonpleuritic and nonpositional. It was not associated with any nausea, vomiting, or dia-phoresis. Nothing he did made the symptoms better or worse. He did not take anything for the symptoms. He stated that the pain waxed and waned for about an hour and went away on its own. He had a similar episode 2

days earlier after eating dinner; however, it did not last as long as his episode today. Both episodes were the same in severity.

He denies having these symptoms prior to his cardiac stent. At that time, his primary symptom was shortness of breath, which he currently denies. After further questioning the patient relates that he has a history of gastroesophageal reflux disease (GERD) and the only other time he has had similar symptoms is with his "reflux"; however, given his cardiac history, he wanted to come in and be sure. Review of medications revealed that the patient has not been taking his omeprazole for 1 week. He was recently started on amlodipine, 5 mg daily, and he was under the impression this medication replaced the omeprazole. When questioned about the absence of ticagrelor or clopidogrel—since he has a history of cardiac stent—he recalls that he took clopidogrel for 2 months after his stent procedure and was told by his cardiologist that he no longer needed anything more than an aspirin after that. Given his cardiovascular history, cardiology has been asked to consult and assist in management further.

## Past Medical History

1. Coronary artery disease (CAD)
2. Hypertension (HTN)
3. Hyperlipidemia (HLD)
4. Type 2 diabetes mellitus (DM)
5. GERD

No history or pulmonary embolus (PE), deep vein thrombosis (DVT), myocardial infarction (MI), or stroke. No thyroid disease, cancer, or lung disease.

## Past Surgical/Procedure History

1. Coronary artery stenting in 2013 (unknown vessel—done at outside hospital)

## Family History

Father: HTN, HLD—deceased

Mother: HTN, HLD—deceased

Sister: HTN, HLD—alive

No children

*Social History*
No tobacco, alcohol, or illicit drugs

*Allergies*
No known drug allergies (NKDA)

*Medications*

1. Amlodipine 5 mg QD (every day)
2. Omeprazole 20 mg QD (has not taken in 1 week)
3. Simvastatin 40 mg QHS (every bedtime)
4. Metformin 500 mg BIDAC (twice daily before meals)
5. Aspirin 81mg QD
6. HCTZ 25 mg QD
7. Metoprolol XL 50 mg BID (twice daily)

*Review of Systems*
Patient reports chest pain and burning as per HPI. No shortness of breath, dizziness, lightheadedness, nausea, vomiting, or diaphoresis. No syncope or near syncope. No palpitations. No orthopnea, paroxysmal nocturnal dyspnea (PND), weight gain or weight loss. No melena, hematochezia, dysuria, or hematuria.

*Physical Exam*
Vital signs:

Blood pressure: left arm 140/78 mmHg; right arm 138/80 mmHg

Pulse: 70 beats per minute

Respirations: 14 breaths per minute

Oxygen saturation: 99% on room air

Temperature: 36.9°C

General appearance: Slender, well-nourished, and well-developed AA male.

Head and neck: Head is normocephalic and atraumatic, without evidence of lesions or masses. Sclera are anicteric. Neck is soft and supple, without thyromegaly or lymphadenopathy.

Cardiac exam: No elevation of jugular venous pressure. No carotid bruits. No abdominal or femoral bruits. Carotid upstroke is brisk. Peripheral pulses are palpable and symmetric. Auscultation of the heart reveals a regular rate and rhythm, S1 and S2 present. No S3 or S4. No murmurs, rubs, heaves, or lifts. Chest wall is nontender to palpation.

Lungs: Clear breath sounds bilaterally with symmetric expansion.

Abdomen: Soft, nontender. Bowel sounds present in all four quadrants. No hepatosplenomegaly. No hepatojugular reflux.

Extremities: Warm and dry. No evidence of edema, clubbing, or cyanosis.

Neurological: Alert and oriented ×3. Cranial nerves are intact. Motor strength is symmetric in bilateral upper and lower extremities. Sensation is intact. No focal neurological deficits.

### Labs/Data

ECG: Normal sinus rhythm. No ST–T-wave abnormalities. No ischemia or infarct.

Chest film: No evidence of infection/inflammation or pulmonary edema.

Labs: Hemoglobin (Hgb) 14.5, hematocrit (Hct) 41.2, white blood cell count (WBC) 4.5, platelets 280,000, D-dimer 0.42, troponin I <0.01, sodium (Na) 140, potassium (K) 3.9, blood urea nitrogen (BUN) 13, creatinine 0.9.

### Impression

This is a 69-year-old AA male with multiple cardiovascular risk factors who presents with chest pain, burning, and the following issues:

1. Chest pain with known history of CAD
2. GERD
3. HTN
4. HLD
5. DM 2

### Plan

1. This patient's chest pain is most consistent with an exacerbation of his GERD. His objective data are negative for any signs of ischemia, and symptoms are not consistent with ischemia. He should be restarted on omeprazole. Follow-up

will be scheduled with his primary care physician in 1 week. Consider outpatient stress testing if symptoms persist. Return to emergency department for any worsening or change in symptoms.

2. Resume omeprazole. Monitor for symptoms. Follow up as stated.

3. Continue current blood pressure medications. Asked patient to keep blood pressure log at home to assess average.

4. Continue statin therapy. Assess liver function tests as well as lipid panel as outpatient every 3 months.

5. Continue metformin. Check glycosylated hemoglobin as outpatient if not done in last 3 months.

*Disposition*
Stable for discharge from the emergency department with the above plan.

## SAMPLE WRITE-UP 2: CONSULT (Chapter 4 Case Scenario)

*Reason for Consult*
Shortness of breath

*History of Present Illness*
A 67-year-old White male with a history of HLD and a recent diagnosis of stage 2 diffuse large B-cell (DLBCL) non-Hodgkin's was admitted yesterday for neutropenic fever. He completed his first cycle of R-CHOP (rituximab, cyclophosphamide, doxorubicin, vincristine, and prednisone) 12 days ago. He additionally had evidence of bilateral pleural effusions and ankle edema, which has been present for the past 4 days. He was started on empiric antibiotic therapy and given a dose of furosemide, 20 mg IV, upon arrival and despite adequate urine output initially has had no improvement in his symptoms and notices a decrease in urinary frequency presently.

Today he developed shortness of breath, described as a feeling of fullness and inability to get air, shortly after breakfast. He feels short of breath at rest and feels more comfortable in the upright position. He noted he was lightheaded with ambulation and has been mildly short of breath for the past few weeks with exertion only. He denies any chest pain, pressure, tightness, or any chest-related symptoms. He denies any nausea, vomiting, diaphoresis, syncope, near syncope, cough, or palpitations. He has had a decline in his blood pressure and is now tachycardic. He has never had a history of heart attack, heart failure, or a blood clot to the lungs.

Initial evaluation by the primary service was concerning for acute heart failure. Chest film was unchanged from admission and notable for cardiomegaly. There is concern he may have developed a chemo-induced cardiomyopathy and, due to his low blood pressure with the possible need for further diuresis, cardiology has been asked to assist in management.

*Past Medical History*

1.  Stage 2 DLBCL
2.  HLD

No history of MI or stroke. No history of PE, DVT, DM, or thyroid problems.

*Past Surgical/Procedure History*

1.  Lymph node biopsies
2.  Tonsillectomy as a child

*Family History*
Unremarkable

*Social History*
No tobacco, alcohol, or illicit drugs

*Allergies*
NKDA

*Medications*

1.  Atorvastatin 40 mg QHS
2.  Heparin 5,000 SQ Q 12 hour
3.  Omeprazole 20 mg QD
4.  Piperacillin/tazobactam 4.5 g IV Q 6 hour

*Review of Systems*
As detailed in HPI. No syncope or near syncope. No palpitations, nausea, vomiting, or diaphoresis. No dizziness. He denies melena, hematochezia, dysuria, or hematuria.

*Physical Exam*
Vital signs:

Blood pressure: Right arm 90/54 mm/Hg; left arm 88/56 mm/Hg

Pulse: 101-109 beats per minute

Respirations: 20 breaths per minute

Oxygen saturation: 95% on 2 L/min $O_2$

Temperature: 36.5°C.

Pulsus paradoxus of 36 mm/Hg

General appearance: Thin-appearing White male in a moderate amount of distress.

Head and neck: Head is normocephalic and atraumatic, without evidence of lesions or masses. Sclera are anicteric. Neck is soft and supple, without thyromegaly. Supraclavicular and cervical lymphadenopathy is present.

Cardiac exam: Jugular venous pressure is elevated to the level of the earlobe. No carotid bruits. No abdominal or femoral bruits. Peripheral pulses are palpable and symmetric. Loss of peripheral pulse is noted on inspiration. Auscultation of the heart reveals distant heart sounds, S1 and S2 present. No S3 or S4. No murmurs, heaves, rubs, or lifts. Chest wall is nontender to palpation.

Lungs: Reduced sounds in bases bilaterally with faint crackles. Symmetric expansion.

Abdomen: Soft, nontender. Bowel sounds present in all four quadrants.

Extremities: Skin cool but dry. There is 2+ pitting edema noted bilaterally in the pretibial and ankle regions. No clubbing or cyanosis.

Neurological: Alert and oriented ×3. Cranial nerves are intact. Motor strength is symmetric in bilateral upper and lower extremities. Sensation is intact. No focal neurological deficits.

*Labs/Data*

    Echo 2 months ago: ejection fraction (EF) 66% with tiny pericardial effusion. Normal right ventricle (RV) size and function. No valvular abnormalities.

    ECG: Sinus tachycardia. Low voltage with evidence of electrical alternans. No ST–T-wave abnormalities. Changes new from prior study.

    Chest film: Bilateral pleural effusions with cardiomegaly noted. Globular appearance of the heart. Bilateral hilar lymphadenopathy.

    Labs: Hgb 9.6, Hct 31, WBC 1,078, platelets 76,000, brain natriuretic peptide (BNP) 98, Na 136, K 4.1, BUN 15, creatinine 1.4.

*Impression*

This is a 67-year-old White male with stage 2 DLBCL being treated for neutropenic fever with mild volume overload who developed shortness of breath with hypotension concerning for heart failure or possibly chemo-induced cardiomyopathy and the following issues:

1.  Shortness of breath—probable tamponade

2.  Stage 2 DLBCL

3.  HLD

*Recommendations*

1.  His shortness of breath is concerning for enlarging pericardial effusion now with tamponade physiology on bedside exam. This was likely well tolerated until diuresis, which has caused RV collapse. Recommend 1 L of normal saline to be infused rapidly. Stat echocardiogram at bedside. If tamponade is confirmed will need urgent pericardiocentis with drain. Fluid should be sent for cytology and culture. Continue supportive measures with fluid and oxygen until treatment.

2.  Management per hematology/oncology team. If pericardial fluid is malignant, may need consideration of pericardial window as it is likely to recur.

3.  Continue statin therapy.

Thank you for the consult. Further recommendations will be added as more data become available.

## SAMPLE WRITE-UP 3: H&P (Chapter 7 Case Scenario)

*Chief Complaint*
ST elevation myocardial infarction (STEMI) alert

*History of Present Illness*
A 62-year-old White female with a history of HTN presented to the emergency department around 1 p.m. with complaints of substernal chest pain and pressure that had started around 11 a.m. She reports profound emotional distress due to the fact her husband died 2 days ago in a car accident. She awoke this morning with vague nausea and noticed the chest pressure beginning around 11 a.m. as she was discussing funeral arrangements with her family. She thought it was anxiety, but the pain persisted without relief so her family brought her to the emergency department for further evaluation and treatment.

The chest pressure is centrally located, nonradiating, nonpositional, and nonpleuritic in nature. She denies any associated dizziness, lightheadedness, palpitations, syncope or near syncope. She denies any shortness of breath or vomiting. She has never experienced pain like this before.

On arrival to the emergency department, vital signs were stable, but ECG showed ST-segment elevation in leads V3–V5. The STEMI alert was activated. It was confirmed that she had no history of bleeding disorders or active bleeding issues. She was not taking any blood thinners or antiplatelet agents. The patient was then given guideline-directed therapy with heparin; ticagrelor, 180 mg; chewable aspirin, 324 mg; and nitroglycerin sublingual. She was taken urgently for coronary angiography.

*Past Medical History*

1. HTN

No history of MI, stroke, PE, DM, or stroke. No lung disease, cancers, or thyroid problems.

*Past Surgical/Procedure History*
Unremarkable

*Family History*
Mother: Ovarian cancer—deceased in her 60s
Father: HTN, kidney disease, and HLD—alive at 87

*Social History*
No tobacco. She drinks an occasional glass of wine with dinner. No illicit drug use.

Husband recently died in car accident.

*Allergies*
NKDA

*Medications*

1.  Lisinopril 10 mg QD

*Review of System*
As per HPI. No cough, orthopnea, PND, weight gain, or weight loss. No decline in functional status recently. No shortness of breath, nausea, vomiting, syncope, or near syncope. No palpitations. Significant emotional stress reported.

*Physical Exam*
Vital signs:

Blood pressure: Right arm 143/74 mmHg, left arm 146/80 mmHg

Pulse: 78 beats per minute

Respirations: 16 breaths per minute

Oxygen saturation: 97% on room air

Temperature: 37.1°C

General appearance: Well-nourished, well-developed White female. Mild distress.

Head and neck: Head is normocephalic and atraumatic, without evidence of lesions or masses. Sclera are anicteric. Neck is soft and supple, without thyromegaly or lymphadenopathy.

Cardiac exam: There is no elevation of jugular venous pressure. No carotid bruits. No abdominal or femoral bruits. Peripheral pulses are palpable and symmetric. Auscultation of the heart reveals a regular rate and rhythm, S1 and S2 present. No S3 or S4. No murmurs, heaves, rubs, or lifts. Chest wall is nontender to palpation.

Lungs: Clear lung sounds bilaterally. Symmetric expansion.

Abdomen: Soft, nontender. Bowel sounds present in all four quadrants.

Extremities: Skin warm and dry. No edema, clubbing, or cyanosis.

eurological: Alert and oriented ×3. Cranial nerves are intact. Motor strength is symmetric in bilateral upper and lower extremities. Sensation is intact. No focal neurological deficits.

## Labs/Data

ECG: Anterior ST-segment elevation noted in leads V3–V5. Normal sinus rhythm.

Chest film: No acute findings. No edema or infection.

Labs: Hgb 12.4, Hct 38, WBC 7,000, Na 141, K 3.9, BUN 10, creatinine 0.7, troponin I 0.39 ng/mL.

Coronary angiography: No obstructive CAD. Left ventriculogram showed apical ballooning.

Echocardiogram: EF 35% with apical akinesis consistent with stress-induced or Takotsubo cardiomyopathy.

## Impression

This is a 62-year-old White female with a history of hypertension and recent profound emotional stress who presented to the emergency department with complaints of chest pressure and evidence of an anterior STEMI on ECG and who underwent urgent coronary angiography with the resultant issues:

1. Takotsubo cardiomyopathy
2. HTN

## Plan

1.  Admit to cardiology. Stress-induced cardiomyopathy likely a result of emotional stress of husband's death. Patient was given guideline-directed therapy for STEMI initially. No need to continue ticagrelor in light of diagnosis. Continue aspirin 81 mg daily. Continue lisinopril. Start metoprolol 25 mg BID. Check lipid panel from blood in lab and add atorvastatin 40 mg QHS. Trend troponin levels until peak. Follow-up visit with repeat echocardiogram in 2 to 3 weeks.

2.  Continue lisinopril, add low-dose beta blocker. Monitor for hypotension.

## Disposition

Full code. Continue observation for 24 to 48 hours.

## SAMPLE WRITE-UP 4: H&P (Chapter 10 Case Scenario)

*Chief Complaint*
Cough

*History of Present Illness*
An 80-year-old obese White male with a past medical history of chronic obstructive pulmonary disorder (COPD), CAD, atrial fibrillation, HTN, HLD, and type 2 DM presented to the emergency department today with a complaint of a dry hacking cough of 1 month's duration. The cough is nonproductive and different from the occasional productive cough he experiences with COPD. He denies any associated fevers or illness, or symptoms of illness. He initially used his inhaler but had no relief of symptoms. He sought treatment at his family doctor after 1 week of symptoms. He was treated for a COPD exacerbation, but reports that he never felt any improvement.

He states the cough comes on primarily when he is lying flat, requiring him to sleep in a recliner during the night for relief. He denies any other associated symptoms such as shortness of breath worse than his baseline, palpitations, chest pain, nausea, vomiting, or syncope or near syncope. He has not had any bleeding issues while taking warfarin for his atrial fibrillation.

Of note he has had increased salt intake over the last few weeks in his daughter's absence with instant meals and soups. He denies any changes in weight or swelling but does note his blood pressure has been elevated during this time frame as well. He has not noticed an increase in heart rate or symptoms consistent with his atrial fibrillation. He is compliant with his continuous positive airway pressure (CPAP) machine. He feels tired from his lack of sleep and spends the majority of his day sitting in his recliner. There is concern he may have mild heart failure; therefore, cardiology has been asked to assist in management.

*Past Medical History*

1.  COPD
2.  HTN
3.  Atrial fibrillation
4.  HLD
5.  DM 2
6.  Obstructive sleep apnea (OSA)

No history of MI, stroke, PE, DVT, or heart failure. No history of cancer or thyroid disorders.

*Past Surgical History*

1. Cholecystectomy
2. Tonsillectomy
3. Ventral hernia repair

*Family History*
Noncontributory

*Social History*
Widowed. Retired from the Navy. Daughter helps with meals but has been out of town.

Former 30-pack per year smoking history. Did drink alcohol while in the Navy—none now.

No illicit drugs.

*Allergies*
NKDA

*Medications*

1. Warfarin 2.5 mg QD
2. Diltiazem XT 120 mg QD
3. Aspirin 81 mg QD
4. Atorvastatin 80 mg QHS
5. Metformin 1,000 mg BID
6. Fluticasone/salmeterol 250/50 mcg
7. Multivitamin QD

*Review of Systems*
As per HPI. Denies chest pain, palpitations, nausea, vomiting, diaphoresis, dizziness, syncope or near syncope. No fever or chills. No melena, hematochezia, dysuria, or hematuria.

*Physical Exam*
Vital Signs:
   Blood pressure: Left arm 166/80 mmHg, right arm 172/82 mmHg

Pulse: 78 beats per minute

Respirations: 16 breaths per minute

Oxygen saturation: 95% on room air

Temperature: 36.6°C

General appearance: Well-nourished, morbidly obese White male in no acute distress.

Head and neck: Head is normocephalic and atraumatic, without evidence of lesions or masses. Sclera are anicteric. Neck is soft and supple, without thyromegaly or lymphadenopathy.

Cardiac Exam: Assessment of jugular veins is difficult due to body habitus. There is elevation of jugular venous pressure to approximately 10 cm $H_2O$. No carotid bruits. No femoral or abdominal bruits. Carotid upstrokes are symmetric and brisk. Peripheral pulses are palpable and symmetric. Auscultation of the heart reveals distant heart tones, a regular rate and rhythm S1 and S2 present, soft S4. No murmurs or rubs. Chest wall is nontender to palpation.

Lungs: Diminished breath sounds bilaterally in bases with scattered crackles primarily in lower lobes bilaterally. Diffuse inspiratory and expiratory wheezing noted anteriorly in bilateral lungs. Symmetric expansion noted.

Abdomen: Obese. Nontender. Bowel sounds present in all four quadrants. No hepatosplenomegaly. No hepatojugular reflux.

Extremities: Warm and dry. 2+ edema in bilateral ankles. 3–4+ massive scrotal edema noted with 4+ pitting edema in the sacrum and posterior thighs. No clubbing or cyanosis.

Neurological: Alert and oriented ×3. Cranial nerves are intact. Motor strength is symmetric in bilateral upper and lower extremities. No focal neurological deficits.

### Labs/Data

ECG: Normal sinus rhythm. No ST–T-wave abnormalities.

Chest film: Bilateral pleural effusions and pulmonary edema.

Labs: Hgb 15, Hct 44, WBC 10,000, platelets 320,000, Na 137, K 4.3, BUN 12, creatinine 1.0, international normalized ratio (INR) 2.2, troponin I <0.01 ng/mL, BNP 269 pg/mL.

*Impression*

This is an 80-year-old obese White male with multiple medical issues who presented to the emergency department with complaints of persistent cough and the following issues:

1. Cough with evidence of new-onset, moderate heart failure
2. COPD
3. Paroxysmal atrial fibrillation
4. HTN
5. HLD
6. DM 2
7. OSA
8. Obesity

*Plan*

1. Admit to cardiology for new-onset heart failure. Obtain echocardiogram to assess left ventricular function. Diurese with IV furosemide with net negative goal of 1 L/d. Maintain strict intake and output with daily standing weights. Fluid restriction of 1,500 mL/d. Low-salt diet. Check daily electrolytes. Convert to oral diuretics once euvolemia is established.
2. Continue current medication for COPD. Nebulizers as needed. Continuous oxygen saturations.
3. Continue warfarin therapy. Check INR daily.
4. Continue current medication for HTN. If EF is low, consider an alternative to diltiazem. Monitor for hypotension with diuresis.
5. Check lipid panel. Continue current statin therapy and adjust if needed based on results.
6. Hold oral diabetic medication and use sliding scale insulin while in hospital.
7. Continue CPAP at HS for OSA.
8. Nutrition consult and heart failure education.

*Disposition*

Full code. Continue inpatient hospital care until adequate diuresis is achieved.

# INDEX

Printed in the United States
By Bookmasters